T0226408

Sports Medicine

Editor

PETER J. CAREK

PRIMARY CARE:
CLINICS IN OFFICE PRACTICE

www.primarycare.theclinics.com

Consulting Editor
JOEL J. HEIDELBAUGH

March 2020 • Volume 47 • Number 1

ELSEVIER

1600 John F. Kennedy Boulevard ● Suite 1800 ● Philadelphia, Pennsylvania, 19103-2899

http://www.theclinics.com

PRIMARY CARE: CLINICS IN OFFICE PRACTICE Volume 47, Number 1
March 2020 ISSN 0095-4543, ISBN-13: 978-0-323-77719-3

Editor: Katerina Heidhausen
Developmental Editor: Laura Fisher

Primary Care: Clinics in Office Practice (ISSN: 0095-4543) is published quarterly by Elsevier Inc., 360 Park Avenue South, New York, NY 10010-1710. Months of issue are March, June, September, and December. Periodicals postage paid at New York, NY and additional mailing offices. Subscription prices are $253.00 per year (US individuals), $538.00 (US institutions), $100.00 (US students), $303.00 (Canadian individuals), $609.00 (Canadian institutions), $100.00 (Canadian students), $357.00 (international individuals), $609.00 (international institutions), and $175.00 (international students). Foreign air speed delivery is included in all *Clinics* subscription prices. All prices are subject to change without notice. POSTMASTER: Send address changes to *Primary Care: Clinics in Office Practice*, Elsevier Periodicals Customer Service, 11830 Westline Industrial Drive, St. Louis, MO 63146. Customer Service Health Sciences Division, Subscription Customer Service, 3251 Riverport Lane, Maryland Heights, MO 63043. **Customer Service: 1-800-654-2452 (U.S. and Canada); 314-447-8871 (outside U.S. and Canada). Fax: 314-447-8029. E-mail: journalscustomerservice-usa@elsevier.com (for print support); journalsonlinesupport-usa@elsevier.com (for online support).**

Reprints. For copies of 100 or more, of articles in this publication, please contact the Commercial Reprints Department, Elsevier Inc., 360 Park Avenue South, New York, NY 10010-1710. Tel. 212-633-3874; Fax: 212-633-3820; E-mail: reprints@elsevier.com.

Primary Care: Clinics in Office Practice is covered in *MEDLINE/PubMed (Index Medicus)* and *EMBASE/ Excerpta Medica, Current Contents/Clinical Medicine,* and *ISI/BIOMED.*

Contributors

CONSULTING EDITOR

JOEL J. HEIDELBAUGH, MD, FAAFP, FACG
Clinical Professor, Departments of Family Medicine and Urology, University of Michigan Medical School, Ann Arbor, Michigan; Ypsilanti Health Center, Ypsilanti, Michigan

EDITOR

PETER J. CAREK, MD, MS
C. Sue and Louis C. Murray, Professor and Chair, Department of Community Health and Family Medicine, University of Florida College of Medicine, Gainesville, Florida

AUTHORS

ANDREW W. ALBANO Jr, DO, FAAFP
Vice Chair, Quality and Medical Affairs, Faculty, Department of Family Medicine, Prisma Health, Assistant Professor, University of South Carolina School of Medicine Greenville, Greenville, South Carolina

CESAR ARGUELLES, MD
Assistant Professor, Department of Family and Community Medicine, Southern Illinois University School of Medicine, Quincy, Illinois

BENJAMIN BOSWELL, DO
Assistant Professor, Department or Orthopedic Surgery and Department of Emergency Medicine, Case Western Reserve University School of Medicine, University Hospitals Cleveland, Cleveland, Ohio

SCOTT BRAGG, PharmD
Associate Professor, Department of Family Medicine, College of Medicine, Clinical Pharmacy and Outcomes Sciences, College of Pharmacy, Medical University of South Carolina, Charleston, South Carolina

PETER J. CAREK, MD, MS
C. Sue and Louis C. Murray, Professor and Chair, Department of Community Health and Family Medicine, University of Florida College of Medicine, Gainesville, Florida

STEPHEN M. CAREK, MD, CAQSM
Assistant Professor, Department of Family Medicine, University of South Carolina School of Medicine Greenville, Medical Director, Center for Family Medicine, Greenville, South Carolina

JAMES R. CLUGSTON, MD, MS, CAQSM
Associate Professor, Department of Community Health and Family Medicine and Department of Neurology, Program Director, Sports Medicine Fellowship, Team Physician, University Athletic Association University of Florida, UF Student Health Care Center, Gainesville, Florida

JAMES M. DANIELS, MD, MPH
Professor, Department of Family and Community Medicine, Southern Illinois University School of Medicine, Quincy, Illinois

ALEXEI DeCASTRO, MD
Associate Professor, Trident/MUSC Family Medicine Residency Program Director, Department of Family Medicine, College of Medicine, Medical University of South Carolina, Charleston, South Carolina

WILLIAM H. DIXON, MD
Assistant Professor, Department of Family and Community Medicine, Southern Illinois University School of Medicine, Quincy, Illinois

JONATHAN A. DREZNER, MD
Department of Family Medicine, UW Medicine Center for Sports Cardiology, University of Washington, Seattle, Washington

KATHERINE M. EDENFIELD, MD
Clinical Assistant Professor, Department of Community Health and Family Medicine, University of Florida, Student Health Care Center, Gainesville, Florida

BENJAMIN FERRY, MD
PGY-3 Resident Physician, Trident/MUSC Family Medicine Residency Program, Department of Family Medicine, Medical University of South Carolina, Charleston, South Carolina

MICHELLE FUTRELL, MA, ATC, SCAT
Director of Center for Academic Performance and Persistence, Senior Instructor, Department of Health and Human Performance, Gallup Certified Strengths Coach and Certified Strengths-Based Education Facilitator (F-CSBE), College of Charleston, Charleston, South Carolina

CHRISTOPHER GLEASON, MD
Associate Professor, Department of Family and Community Medicine, Southern Illinois University School of Medicine, Springfield, Illinois

VICKI NELSON, MD, PhD
Assistant Professor, University of South Carolina School of Medicine Greenville, Faculty, Department of Family Medicine, Prisma Health, Greenville, South Carolina

BENJAMIN OSHLAG, MD
Assistant Professor, Department of Emergency Medicine, Icahn School of Medicine at Mount Sinai, Mount Sinai Beth Israel Hospital, New York, New York

TRACY RAY, MD
Associate Professor, Department of Family Medicine and Department of Orthopedic Surgery, Duke University, Durham, North Carolina

LISA K. ROLLINS, PhD
Associate Professor, Department of Family Medicine, Director, Faculty Development Fellowship, University of Virginia Health System, Charlottesville, Virginia

SUSAN L. ROZZI, PhD, ATC, SCAT
Associate Professor, Department of Health and Human Performance, Faculty Fellow, Center for Academic Performance and Persistence, College of Charleston, Charleston, South Carolina

DAVID M. SIEBERT, MD
Department of Family Medicine, UW Medicine Center for Sports Cardiology, University of Washington, Seattle, Washington

SIOBHAN M. STATUTA, MD
Director, Primary Care Sports Medicine Fellowship, Associate Professor, Departments of Family Medicine, Physical Medicine and Rehabilitation, Team Physician, University of Virginia Sports Medicine, University of Virginia Health System, Charlottesville, Virginia

COLTON L. WOOD, MD
Resident Physician, PGY-3, Department of Family Medicine, University of Virginia Health System, Charlottesville, Virginia

Contents

Although the specific content has been recommended, debated, and extensively reviewed over the past several decades, the preparticipation evaluation (PPE) has become standard of care for athletes as they prepare for organized athletic participation. The PPE seeks to detect conditions that predispose the athlete to injury or limit full participation in certain activities. Of particular interest, underlying cardiovascular and musculoskeletal conditions are sought because they are frequently associated with mortality and morbidity in athletes.

Primary care clinicians fulfill critical roles of screening for, diagnosing, and managing cardiovascular disease. In young athletes, primary structural and electrical diseases are the focus. Coronary artery disease is the chief concern in older athletes. Sudden cardiac arrest may be the initial presentation of disease and is more common in young athletes than historically appreciated. The traditional preparticipation evaluation, or sports physical, is limited in its ability to accurately raise suspicion of underlying disease. The 12-lead electrocardiogram is a more accurate screening tool. Contemporary risk stratification and treatment protocols may allow for safe return to sport on a case-by-case basis.

Sports supplements can be generally divided into 3 categories: sports foods (foods/drinks containing macronutrients), medical supplements (vitamins/minerals used to treat deficiencies), and ergogenic supplements (used to benefit performance). Supplements are not regulated by the US Food and Drug Administration. They may get to the market and be contaminated with substances banned in sport or dangerous to health; and the contents may not contain what is listed on the label. When choosing to use a supplement, the safest practice is to choose a certified brand, which tests and authenticates label verification, quality, and lack of contaminants and banned substances for sport.

> Athletes of various skill levels commonly use many different types of medications, often at rates higher than the general population. Common medication classes used in athletes include analgesics such as nonsteroidal anti-inflammatory drugs and acetaminophen, inhalers for asthma and exercise-induced bronchoconstriction, antihypertensives, antibiotics, and insulin. Prescribers must be aware of the unique considerations for each of these medications when using them in patients participating in physical activity. The safety, efficacy, impact on athletic performance, and regulatory restrictions of the most common medications used in athletes are discussed in this article.

> Women are increasingly participating in more and more sporting activities. For years, women athletes have been treated as the "female" equivalent of male athletes, with similar medical approaches but this is changing. The concept that women are unique in their "athletic arena" is further underscored with emerging scientific evidence—from the physiologic details not visible to the eye, to the more overt biomechanical and anatomic differences. We review a handful of conditions active women potentially may encounter: pregnancy, the female athlete triad, patellofemoral pain, potential injuries to the anterior cruciate ligament, and anemia.

> Developing and implementing a rehabilitation program is one of the most challenging patient care skills because it requires a firm grasp of the healing process and available treatment options, which must then be serially compared with the pathologic condition of the injury and the patient's progress. This cyclical problem-based approach to rehabilitation allows clinicians to most effectively individualize the rehabilitation plan to the patient's individual needs and progress. In each phase of the rehabilitation process, problems should be identified and goals developed taking into consideration the phase of healing.

> Primary care and sports medicine physicians will undoubtedly encounter upper-extremity injuries on a regular basis in their practice. Athletes have injuries most commonly to the shoulder, elbow, wrist, and hand as a result of a fall onto an outstretched arm. This article aims to educate physicians about sports-related upper-extremity injuries. Common mechanisms of injury, classic physical examination, and radiographic findings are reviewed. General guidelines for treatment as well as indications for referral to a sports medicine or orthopedic specialist are included in the discussion.

Hip and knee injuries are a common presenting concern for patients to a primary care office. This pathology represents a large differential and it can often be a diagnostic challenge for providers to determine the etiology of a patient's symptoms. This article discusses several of the most common causes for hip and knee pain while providing an evidence based review of physical examination maneuvers, imaging studies and treatment modalities to assist a primary care provider when encountering active patients with underlying hip or knee pain.

Foot and ankle injuries account for a significant volume of primary care office visits each year. Given the incidence of injury and concern for long-term sequelae, it is imperative that primary care physicians familiarize themselves with commonly encountered foot and ankle injuries. Coupling a sound understanding of key anatomic structures with an appropriately gathered history can help to quickly narrow the differential diagnosis in this clinical presentation. This article focuses on key elements from the history and physical examination as well as provides a concise review of imaging modalities and recommended treatment strategies.

When searching for evidence-based answers about treating athletes with low back injury/pain, there are some difficulties. The first is defining who is an athlete. The second problem is that the lifetime prevalence of low back pain in the general population in our country approaches 100. Last, most studies published only deal with a narrow population of athletes, often performing very different types of physical activity. We searched the literature for studies that specifically evaluated athletes longitudinally. This article reviews the demographics, diagnostic challenges, history and physical examination, imaging choices, treatment, and controversies encountered when treating this population.

Neck injuries are relatively uncommon but have the potential to cause serious and permanent disability. In athletes, injuries are most common in contact sports, and occur with direct axial loading with a forward-flexed neck. Soft tissue and peripheral nerve injuries are typically minor and self-limiting, with excellent recovery potential and return to activities based on symptoms. Concern for devastating spinal cord injuries has led to routine immobilization using spine boards and hard cervical collars. This approach may provide more harm than benefit when applied universally, and a more commonsense protocol can be used to better address potential neck injuries.

Injuries from sports-related head trauma are commonly encountered by primary care providers. These injuries vary in clinical presentation, severity, and outcome, with sports-related concussion (SRC) being the most common and more severe sports-related head trauma, such as hemorrhage, and "second impact syndrome" occurring rarely. Understanding the importance of immediate recognition, removal from play, multimodal evaluation, and typical patterns of recovery is necessary to safely manage an athlete with SRC. Proper care of athletes with severe sports-related head trauma requires a high index of suspicion and appropriate initial management to maximize survival and minimize morbidity.

PRIMARY CARE:
CLINICS IN OFFICE PRACTICE

SERIES OF RELATED INTEREST

Clinics in Sports Medicine (http://www.sportsmed.theclinics.com)
Orthopedic Clinics (http://www.orthopedic.theclinics.com)
Medical Clinics (http://www.medical.theclinics.com)

THE CLINICS ARE AVAILABLE ONLINE!
Access your subscription at:
www.theclinics.com

Foreword

Aches and Pains, Goals, and Gains

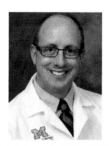

Joel J. Heidelbaugh, MD, FAAFP, FACG
Consulting Editor

Many of us at 1 point or another in our lives have considered ourselves to be athletes, or at least "athletic." Even if we haven't, life is full of activities, chores, and work: all of which create an element of physical stress and strain often when we least expect it. Sore necks and backs abound coupled with the random joint and even foot pain, created by physical activity, sitting at a computer, or something as simple as lifting a laundry basket. One of the most brutal injuries I've sustained in my first half-century of life involved lifting: a sock that I dropped on the floor. Six weeks of left-sided back pain and sciatica made daily life and work nearly untenable. Fortunately, the right diagnostic evaluation and committed therapy allowed me to escape surgery.

Musculoskeletal complaints, aches and pains, and injuries across the spectrum of severity are common in daily primary care practices. Just this morning in clinic alone, I evaluated a very physically fit middle-aged runner who has a partially avulsed hamstring and right ischial tuberosity inflammation, a woman who works on the assembly line at an automotive plant with a torn supraspinatus, and a high school basketball player with chronic Achilles tendinitis, and I detected a new murmur in a 14-year-old otherwise healthy girl who presented for her well adolescent examination and to get clearance to play volleyball. I've had the privilege of caring for athletes ranging from age 4 through high school and collegiate athletes, and even an adult Olympic sprinter. Each patient, sport, and level of competition provide unique opportunities to prepare athletes for training and competition and to help them toward rehabilitation.

While most primary care providers feel confident in their musculoskeletal examinations and diagnostic workups guidelines change, novel treatment modalities create opportunities to allow our patients more expedited recovery. This issue of *Primary Care: Clinics in Office Practice* presents detailed articles that cover the approach and treatment to head, spine, extremity injuries, as well as unique medical concerns in the female athlete. A very interesting article on common supplements that athletes use provides insight into what works and what doesn't, and what should be and what

Prim Care Clin Office Pract 47 (2020) xiii–xiv
https://doi.org/10.1016/j.pop.2019.12.002
0095-4543/20/© 2019 Published by Elsevier Inc.

primarycare.theclinics.com

shouldn't be used. Articles highlighting the preparticipation examination and detection of underlying cardiac conditions provide current evidence-based guidelines. Last, principles of rehabilitation and how to incorporate them into practice allow for additional care that primary care providers can offer, especially as in some cases waiting times to see a physical therapist may be increasing.

My brilliant colleague Dr Peter Carek and his authors are to be commended for creating this outstanding issue of articles on sports medicine and related musculoskeletal topics. Each provides a practical guide to the many elements of this topic that can be readily incorporated into daily practice. What is most unique about this issue is that it can serve as a "how-to" guide to help our patients reach their rehabilitative goals and to make substantial gains in health and strength.

Joel J. Heidelbaugh, MD, FAAFP, FACG
Departments of Family Medicine and Urology
University of Michigan Medical School
Ann Arbor, MI 48103, USA

Ypsilanti Health Center
200 Arnet, Suite 200
Ypsilanti, MI 48198, USA

E-mail address:
jheidel@umich.edu

Preface

Every Patient Seen in Primary Care Is an Athlete (to a Degree)

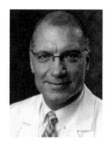

Peter J. Carek, MD, MS
Editor

As primary care physicians, advance practice providers, or other members of the health care team, we recommend physical activity to most if not all patients we see. On a population basis, and most importantly, regular physical activity prevents the development of coronary artery disease and reduces symptoms in patients with established cardiovascular disease. Furthermore, evidence supports the role of exercise in reducing the risk of several other chronic diseases, including type 2 diabetes mellitus, osteoporosis, obesity, and cancer of the breast and colon. As such, we serve directly or indirectly as primary care sports medicine physicians and providers as we routinely care for the physically active patient population we aim to create.

With that said, this issue of *Primary Care: Clinics in Office Practice* is meant to guide you in your care of an active patient population. Whether it be an individual who recently began an exercise program or an athlete involved in organized sport at any level, the topics and conditions addressed in this issue are commonly seen by physicians and other providers primarily providing health care to patients.

As you will see, a broad range of pertinent topics are covered. We begin with a discussion of the preparticipation evaluation and augment this information with a review of the cardiac diseases that impact athletes. If any of your patients are involved in organized sports, the article on the preparticipation examination will be an invaluable resource. Next, we present articles on the use of sports supplements and prescription medications in athletes. An article specific to the female athlete is next and highlights the unique aspects and issues that occur in this specific patient population.

As you treat the physically active patient, you will soon realize the predominant "side effect" of this activity is musculoskeletal complaints, whether acute or chronic. To begin this section, an overview of the principles of rehabilitation is presented. These principles are important to understand as they provide an overall guide and allow you to successfully treat common musculoskeletal conditions. The next 6 articles

Prim Care Clin Office Pract 47 (2020) xv–xvi
https://doi.org/10.1016/j.pop.2019.12.001
0095-4543/20/© 2019 Published by Elsevier Inc.

primarycare.theclinics.com

address injuries to the major areas of the musculoskeletal system commonly affected by regular physical activity: Upper extremity, hip and knee, ankle and foot, back, neck, and head.

The information in this issue is presented by a group of professionals actively involved in serving as primary care physicians as well as primary care sports medicine physicians. As such, they have a unique insight that allows for a thorough and useful presentation of their subject area.

I hope you enjoy this issue and find the content as insightful and useful as I do.

Peter J. Carek, MD, MS
Department of Community Health and Family Medicine
University of Florida College of Medicine
1600 SW Archer Road
MSB N 1-02
PO Box 100237
Gainesville, FL 32610-0237, USA

E-mail address:
carek@ufl.edu

Preparticipation Evaluation

Stephen M. Carek, MD, CAQSM[a], Katherine M. Edenfield, MD[b],
Peter J. Carek, MD, MS[b],*

KEYWORDS

- Preparticipation evaluation • Sudden cardiac death • Noninvasive cardiac screening
- Musculoskeletal injury

KEY POINTS

- Although athletic participation places the individual at risk for acute musculoskeletal injury or worsening of an underlying medical condition, the mortality associated with athletic participation is most often the result of acute sudden cardiac arrest/death.
- A medical history should be obtained from each athlete and has been shown to identify most problems that affect initial athletic participation.
- Because a cardiac pathologic condition is the most common cause of sudden death in the young, athletic population, the cardiovascular examination requires an additional level of detail and standardization.
- The use of noninvasive cardiac testing (eg, electrocardiography, electrocardiography, or exercise stress testing) is an area of significant debate and research and, at present, is not uniformly considered a routine aspect of the screening preparticipation evaluation.

The preparticipation evaluation (PPE) is often a requirement and, in many areas, has become the standard of care for athletes as they prepare for organized athletic participation. This requirement was established because of both medical and legal concerns for athletes that could be at an increased risk for severe injury or death because of participation. The specific content of the PPE has been recommended, debated, and extensively reviewed by numerous authorities in sports medicine over the past several decades.[1–36]

The American Academy of Family Physicians, the American Academy of Pediatrics, the American College of Sports Medicine, the American Medical Society for Sports Medicine, the American Orthopedic Society for Sports Medicine, and the American Osteopathic Academy of Sports Medicine updated the previously published monograph *Preparticipation Physical Evaluation*.[37] The recommendations found in this article serve as a guide for the physician conducting these

[a] Department of Family Medicine, University of South Carolina, School of Medicine–Greenville, Center for Family Medicine - Greenville, 877 West Faris Road, Greenville, SC 29605, USA;
[b] Department of Community Health and Family Medicine, University of Florida College of Medicine, 1600 SW Archer Road, MSB N 1-02, PO Box 100237, Gainesville, FL 32610-0237, USA
* Corresponding author.
E-mail address: carek@ufl.edu

Prim Care Clin Office Pract 47 (2020) 1–17
https://doi.org/10.1016/j.pop.2019.10.001
0095-4543/20/© 2019 Elsevier Inc. All rights reserved.
primarycare.theclinics.com

examinations for their local high school and collegiate athletes. The 2015 *Eligibility and Disqualification Recommendations for Competitive Athletes with Cardiovascular Abnormalities: A Scientific Statement from the American Heart Association and American College of Cardiology* is an update to the 2005 36th Bethesda Conference guidelines,[3] and The European Society of Cardiology guidelines regarding *Pre-participation cardiovascular evaluation for athletic participants to prevent sudden death* contribute various guidelines for athletic preparticipation cardiovascular screening.[38–40]

In the United States, most states and the National Collegiate Athletic Association (NCAA) require a PPE for high school and college student athletes, respectively. Internationally, the PPE varies in frequency of use and content.[32] The Italian government has required screening and medical clearance of all young athletes since 1971. In contrast, the British think widespread population screening is not appropriate, particularly in relation to cardiomyopathy, and maintain that identifying people at risk is vital for effective intervention.[41] Rather than providing a PPE, a process of profiling or ongoing monitoring of player health and performance has been introduced to elite-level athletes in Great Britain.[42] Although validity has yet to be studied, profiling is intended to minimize the incidence of illness, fatigue, and overuse injuries. In Germany, a PPE with electrocardiography (ECG) is recommended for all leisure time athletes and competitive athletes at lower levels. All elite athletes are examined with history and physical examination, ECG, exercise testing, and echocardiography (ECHO).[43] Interestingly, Japan requires ECG screening for all children in school grades 1, 7, and 10, regardless if they participate in organized athletic activity.[44]

In addition to its stated objectives, the PPE appears to serve other purposes (**Box 1**). Several studies have found that many athletes use this examination as their only contact with a health care provider.[45,46] From a provider perspective, mass preparticipation screening events may serve to provide public awareness of a physician's or medical group's interest in providing sports medicine services.

Although the PPE often detects conditions that may predispose the athlete to injury or limit full participation in certain activities, most athletes are cleared during the PPE without significant medical or orthopedic abnormalities being noted. In previous reported results of mass preparticipation screening events, approximately 5% to 15% of athletes require further evaluation; less than 3% fail the examination and are denied participation (**Table 1**).[47–56] These conditions are

---

Box 1
Objectives of the preparticipation physical evaluation

Primary
- Screen for conditions that may be life threatening or disabling.
- Screen for conditions that may predispose to injury or illness.

Secondary
- Determine general health of the individual.
- Serve as an entry point to the health care system.
- Provide an opportunity to initiate discussion on health-related topics.

From Bernhardt DT, Roberts WO, editors. Goals and objectives. In: Preparticipation physical evaluation (4th edition). Elk Grove Village, IL: American Academy of Pediatrics; 2010. p. 7; with permission.

Table 1
Rates of clearance, clearance with a medical condition, or full restriction

	Number of Athletes	Pass (%)	Pass with Condition (%)	Fail (%)
Goldberg et al,[47] 1980	701	85.2	13.5	1.3
Linder et al,[48] 1981	1268	94.8	5.0	0.2
Tennant et al,[49] 1981	2719	89.6	9.2	1.2
Thompson et al,[50] 1982	2670	89.2	9.6	1.2
DuRant et al,[122] 1985	922	94.4	5.6	0.3
Risser et al,[52] 1985	2114	96.6	3.1	0.3
Magnes et al,[53] 1992	10,540	89.4	10.2	0.4
Rifat et al,[54] 1995	2574	84.8	12.6	2.6
Lively,[55] 1999	596	85.9	13.9	0.2
Mayer et al,[56] 2012	733	94.5	5.2	0.4

Data from Refs.[47–56]

usually limited to several organ systems (ie, musculoskeletal and cardiovascular) (**Table 2**).[54,55,57,58]

ATHLETIC MORTALITY AND MORBIDITY

In young individuals (<35 years old), the mortality associated with athletic participation is most often the result of acute sudden cardiac death and occurs with reported incidence that varies between 1 per 23,000 to one in a million athletes per year.[59–61] Certain subpopulations appear to be at more risk, with the highest incidence of 1 per 3100 athletes per year reported in NCAA Division 1 male basketball players.[62] Although a more limited incidence range of 0.5 to 1 per 200,000 athletes per year is often reported, the rate appears to be influenced by numerous factors, including reporting methods, annual variation of events, and variations in populations studied.[62] For instance, the annual incidence of sudden cardiac death in the United States is about 1 in 80,000 in high school athletes and 1 in 50,000 in college athletes.[63]

Athletic participation also places the individual at risk for acute musculoskeletal injury or worsening of an underlying medical condition. In terms of anatomic sites, the most common injury to restrict participation is a knee injury, followed by an ankle injury.[51] The strongest independent predictor of sports injuries is a previous injury (odds ratio [OR] = 9.4) and exposure time (OR = 6.9).[64] DuRant and colleagues[51] found having previously experienced a knee injury or having undergone knee surgery was significantly associated with knee injuries during the subsequent sports season when compared with individuals who did not report previous knee injury or surgery (30.6% vs 7.2%, P = .0001). Many of these acute musculoskeletal injuries may result in long-term health issues (osteoarthritis) that may impact both participation and treatment decisions.

PREPARTICIPATION EVALUATION OF AN ATHLETE
Medical History

A medical history should be obtained from each athlete. A complete medical history has been shown to identify approximately 75% of problems that affect initial athletic

Table 2
Medical and orthopedic conditions found in junior/senior high school (Rifat et al,[54] 1995) and college-aged (Lively,[55] 1999) athletes resulting in additional recommendations

| | Rifat et al,[54] 1995[a] | | Lively,[55] 1999[b] |
| | n = 2574 | | n = 596 |
	Pass with Follow-Up and/or Restriction (12.6%)	Fail with Follow-Up (2.6%)	Follow-Up or Restriction (14.1%)
Medical (% of overall total)	76.6	74.1	55.4
Cardiovascular	18.3	35.0	63.0
Dermatologic	6.8	—	—
Endocrinologic	0.4	—	—
Ears/nose/throat	9.6	2.5	—
Gastrointestinal	0.9	—	2.2
Genitourinary	9.6	12.5	8.7
Gynecologic	—	—	4.4
Infectious	0.4	—	6.5
Neurologic	—	—	6.5
Ophthalmologic	26.0	25.0	6.5
Psychological	—	—	2.2
Pulmonary	14.2	2.5	—
Other[c]	13.7	22.5	—
Total medical (%)	100.0	100.0	100.0
Orthopedic (% of overall total)	23.4	25.9	44.6
Ankle/foot	14.9	7.7	2.7
Back/neck	22.4	14.3	5.4
Elbow	—	—	5.4
Hand/wrist	1.5		10.9
Knee	41.8	7.1	43.2
Leg	—	—	5.4
Shoulder	—	—	27.0
Nonspecific pain/injury	19.4	71.4	—
Total orthopedic (%)	100.0	100.0	100.0

[a] Two individuals failed (nonspecific pain/injury).
[b] One individual failed (complicated pregnancy).
[c] Other includes abdominal pain, allergy, bruising, chest pain, chronic/recurrent illness, dizziness/syncope with exercise, surgery (recent).

participation and serves as the foundation of the PPE.[37,47,52] Unfortunately, these studies noted that the sensitivity of the recommended questionnaires is approximately 50%, below the usual standard expected from a medical screening test.

Most conditions requiring further evaluation or restriction have been reported to be identified during this aspect of the evaluation process. In an earlier study, Rifat and colleagues[54] noted that the history accounted for 88% of the abnormal findings and 57% of the reasons cited for activity restriction. The Preparticipation Physical

Evaluation Task Force has developed a history form that emphasizes the areas of greatest concern for sports participation.[37] In 2014, the American College of Cardiology and American Heart Association (AHA) jointly released recommendations for congenital and genetic heart disease screenings in youth that included a 14-element screening checklist (**Box 2**).[65] A positive response to any of these questions requires confirmation and further evaluation, although a normal history does not exclude underlying cardiac pathologic condition.

Additional historical information needs to be included.[37] For example, the athlete should be questioned about the presence of wheezing during exercise. Because of the high rate of recurrence and potential for long-term adverse effects, a history of previous concussions should be obtained. Other issues to be addressed should include presence of a single bilateral organ in athletes participating in sports with high risk to the remaining organ and use of performance-enhancing medication. Finally, female athletes should be questioned regarding their menstrual history and other symptoms or signs of energy deficiency that could affect bone health and performance.[66,67]

The recommendations by the PPE task force and others have included questions regarding lifestyle choices and preventive services not previously recommended for

---

Box 2
American Heart Association 14-element screening checklist

Medical history (parental verification recommended for high school and middle school athletes)

Personal history
1. Exertional chest pain/discomfort
2. Exertional syncope or near syncope[a]
3. Excessive exertional and unexplained fatigue/fatigue associated with exercise
4. Prior recognition of a heart murmur
5. Elevated systemic blood pressure
6. Prior restriction from participation in sports
7. Prior testing for the heart ordered by a physician

Family history
8. Premature death, sudden and unexpected before age 50 years due to heart disease, in one or more relatives
9. Disability from heart disease in a close relative less than 50 years old
10. Specific knowledge of certain cardiac conditions in family members: hypertrophic or dilated cardiomyopathy, long-QT syndrome or other ion channelopathies, Marfan syndrome, or clinically important arrhythmias

Physical examination
11. Heart murmur[b]
12. Femoral pulses to exclude aortic stenosis
13. Physical stigmata of Marfan syndrome
14. Brachial artery blood pressure (sitting, preferably taken in both arms)

[a] Judged not to be of neurocardiogenic (vasovagal) origin, of particular concern when occurring during or after physical exertion.
[b] Refers to heart murmurs judged likely to be organic and unlikely to be innocent; auscultation should be performed with the patient in both the supine and standing positions (or with Valsalva maneuver), specifically to identify murmurs of dynamic left ventricular outflow tract obstruction.
From Maron BJ, Friedman RA, Kligfield P, et al. Assessment of the 12-lead ECG as a screening test for detection of cardiovascular disease in healthy general populations of young people (12-25 years of age). J Am Coll Cardiol 2014;64(14):1482; with permission.

this particular examination.[37] Although most athletes think that the PPE prevents or helps to prevent injuries, no clear evidence is present to support this assumption, and athletes are not consistently receptive to some preventive health screening.[46] For example, some athletes do not feel comfortable with certain issues being raised (ie, gynecologic health, eating disorders, alcohol and nicotine use).

The historical information provided by the athlete and their parent should be reviewed carefully and additional questions used to clarify any discrepancies. In 2 separate studies, minimal agreement was found between histories obtained from athletes and parents independently.[52,68] Of particular note, unreliable information may be obtained regarding cardiovascular and musculoskeletal issues.[68] Both the parents and the student athlete should be questioned and specific answers confirmed because the source that provides the most accurate history is not clear.

Physical Examination

For the PPE, a limited physical examination is recommended. The screening physical examination should include vital signs (ie, height, weight, and blood pressure) and visual acuity testing as well as a cardiovascular, pulmonary, abdominal, skin, and musculoskeletal examination. Further examination should be based on issues elicited during the history.

Because a cardiac pathologic condition is the most common cause of sudden death in the young, athletic population, the cardiovascular examination requires an additional level of detail and standardization. Auscultation of the heart is performed initially with the patient in both standing and supine position. Auscultation must also occur during at least 2 maneuvers (ie, squat-to-stand, deep inspiration, or Valsalva maneuver) because these maneuvers may clarify the type of murmur. Any systolic murmur grade III/VI or louder, any murmur that disrupts normal heart sounds, any diastolic murmur, or any murmur that intensifies with the previously described maneuvers should be evaluated further through diagnostic studies (eg, ECG or ECHO) or consultation before participation. Sinus bradycardia and systolic murmurs are commonly found, occurring in more than 50% and between 30% to 50% of athletes, respectively, and do not warrant further evaluation in the asymptomatic athlete.[69] Third and fourth heart sounds are also commonly found in asymptomatic athletes without underlying heart disease.[69,70] In addition, it is important to identify and classify normal and abnormal blood pressure values for pediatric athletes using appropriate age-, gender-, and height-based tables.

The screening musculoskeletal examination is also an integral aspect of the PPE and a source for further evaluations, referrals, interventions, and follow-up. A screening musculoskeletal history and examination in combination can be used for asymptomatic athletes with no previous injuries (**Table 3**).[71] An accurate history is able to detect more than 90% of significant musculoskeletal injuries. The screening physical examination is 51% sensitive and 97% specific.[71] If the athlete has either a previous injury or other signs or symptoms (ie, pain, tenderness, asymmetries in muscle bulk, strength, or range of motion, and any obvious deformity) detected by the general screening examination or history, the general screen should be supplemented with relevant elements of an anatomic site-specific examination.

Additional forms of musculoskeletal evaluation are often performed for athletes to determine their general state of flexibility and muscular strength. Although various degrees of hyperlaxity, muscular tightness, weakness, asymmetry of strength or flexibility, poor endurance, and abnormal foot configuration may predispose an athlete to increased risk of injury during sports competition, the studies have failed

Table 3
The "90-second" musculoskeletal screening examination

Instruction	Observations
Stand facing examiner	Acromioclavicular joints: general habitus
Look at ceiling, floor, over both shoulders touch ears to shoulder	Cervical spine motion
Shrug shoulders (resistance)	Trapezius strength
Abduct shoulders to 90° (resistance at 90°)	Deltoid strength
Full external rotation of arms	Shoulder motion
Flex and extend elbows	Elbow motion
Arms at sides, elbows at 90° flexed; pronate and supinate wrists	Elbow and wrist motion
Spread fingers; make fist	Hand and finger motion, strength, and deformities
Tighten (contract) quadriceps; relax quadriceps	Symmetry and knee effusions, ankle effusion
"Duck walk" away and toward examiner	Hip, knee, and ankle motions
Back to examiner	Shoulder symmetry; scoliosis
Knees straight, touch toes	Scoliosis, hip motion, hamstring tightness
Raise up on toes, heels	Calf symmetry, leg strength

to demonstrate conclusively that injuries are prevented by interventions aimed at correcting such abnormalities.[72–75] Meeuwisse and Fowler[76] reported that new injuries were found to have no relationship to previous injury, flexibility, range of motion, strength, or other factors identifiable on preseason musculoskeletal examination.

As noted by Garrick,[77] little if any evidence exists regarding the premise that any level of loss of motion or strength is predictive of an increased likelihood of subsequent injury. In addition, evidence that stretching to increase range of motion prevents injury is lacking. In a systematic review to assess the evidence for the effectiveness of stretching as a tool to prevent injuries in sports, stretching was not significantly associated with a reduction in total injuries.[78] In addition, the findings of musculoskeletal screening may lead to additional testing (eg, radiographic studies) and interventions (eg, physical therapy, orthotics) with unclear benefit for the athlete. Smith and Laskowski[79] noted that the absence of concrete recommendations concerning the findings from a preparticipation screening examination is attributable to the lack of consensus regarding the threshold for abnormality, the unavailability of data indicating the predictive value of specific physical abnormalities for injury, and the lack definitive proof that corrective interventions alter outcome.

The remainder of the physical examination may be limited to the following anatomic areas: general appearance, eyes/ears/nose/throat, lymph nodes, lungs, and abdomen. Any abnormalities in these areas should be further investigated. Of particular interest and often discomfort for the athlete is the male genitalia examination, mainly attempting to identify the presence of an inguinal hernia. The effectiveness of this partial examination in identifying asymptomatic conditions that require further evaluation and potential treatment or that restrict an individual from athletic participation is unclear and not well studied. In terms of asymptomatic or minimally symptomatic inguinal hernias, no treatment is indicated, suggesting a screening question may be sufficient.[80]

Noninvasive Cardiac Testing

The use of noninvasive cardiac testing (eg, ECG, ECHO, or exercise stress testing) is an area of significant debate and research. At present, these tests are not uniformly considered a routine aspect of the screening PPE.[37] Previous studies did not find that these studies were cost-effective in a population at relatively low risk for cardiac abnormalities and cannot consistently identify athletes at actual risk.[81–85] Recently, the sensitivity and specificity of athlete ECG interpretation have been improved if appropriate athlete-specific criteria are used.[61] Despite the tools available, the AHA does not recommend universal mandatory ECG screening of athletes.[65]

A benefit of an initial cardiovascular screening protocol that included family and personal history, physical examination, basal 12-lead ECG, and limited exercise testing was reported.[86] In this study, the sudden death rate among athletes in the prescreening period was reduced from 3.6 per 100,000 person-years in the prescreening period to 0.4 per 100,000 person-years at the end of the study. In a subsequent study using similar screening methods, mandatory ECG screening of athletes had no effect on their risk for cardiac arrest despite the incidence of sudden death of athletes in the study within a similar range as reported by others.[87] These investigators concluded that the findings in the Italian study were secondary to large year-to-year variations.

Screening for predisposing conditions is difficult and limited by several coexisting issues: the low prevalence of cardiovascular diseases responsible for sudden death (SD) in the young population, the low risk of SD among those with the diseases, the large sizes of the populations proposed for screening, and the imperfection of the 12-lead ECG as a screening or diagnostic tool in this setting.[65]

A valid concern with ECG screening is the potential for costly second-tier follow-up testing (eg, ECHOs and MRI) while only detecting rare true-positive results.[38,87–89] However, even if ECGs with false-positive results could be reduced to only 5% in the course of screening 10 million individuals (the estimated number of US competitive athletes), screening ECGs would nevertheless identify a formidable obstacle of 500,000 people who required further testing to exclude underlying heart disease and resolve eligibility for sports participants. Very few of these individuals would ultimately prove to have important disease with a risk for SD that required disqualification.[65]

Unfortunately, the common cardiac conditions that limit athletic participation and contribute to athletic mortality are nearly never detected during the PPE. The most prevalent congenital heart diseases (ventricular septal defect, atrial septal defect, patent ductus arteriosis, pulmonic stenosis, and aortic stenosis) are generally recognized early in life and are therefore unlikely to be first detected during the preparticipation process.[90] Many cardiomyopathies causing sudden cardiac death are not detected during screening because ECG and ECHO were not sensitive enough to detect disease.[91] Maron and colleagues[92] identified that upwards of 70% of cardiovascular sudden death was undetected despite normal screening history, physical examination, and ECG.

Certain populations of athletes appear to be at higher risk for sudden cardiac death.[32] For instance, 4 sports (American football, basketball, track, and soccer) are associated with most of the sudden deaths. In addition, approximately 90% of athletic-field deaths have occurred in male athletes, and most of the individuals affected were high school athletes.[65,92,93] In addition, NCAA black male athletes, and in particular, NCAA Division 1 basketball male athletes of any ethnicity, have among the highest relative risk.[93] This finding lends some institutions to consider more specific cardiovascular screening for those populations at higher risk.

The prevalence of underlying cardiovascular disease varies according to ethnic background and nationality. The Brugada syndrome in which right bundle branch block with persistent ST segment elevation in the right precordial leads is associated with susceptibility to ventricular tachyarrhythmias, and sudden cardiac death is more prevalent in those of Asian descent.[94] Although hypertrophic cardiomyopathy is found to be the most common cause of sudden death in athletes in the United States, arrhythmogenic right ventricular dysplasia is the most common cause of sudden death among Italian athletes.[95] More recent studies in NCAA athletes have shown autopsy-negative sudden death (presumed to be arrhythmia related) to be the most common cause of cardiac death, with cardiomyopathies being the second most common cause.[96]

Presently, the use of a screening ECG as part of the PPE remains controversial and an area requiring further research.[97–99] The impact of ECG screening for truly asymptomatic individuals before athletic participation is not clearly known, and the decision to use ECG screening should be based on individual circumstances.

Although the value of a screening ECG to prevent acute sudden cardiac death in athletes is yet to be determined, certain information and specific criteria are present that will assist physicians who do use the ECG as a screening tool. First, the screening ECG increases the detection of cardiac disorders in athletes.[100] Second, the results of screening ECG should not be used to exclude individuals for further monitoring or evaluation because of the known false negative rate. Finally, specific criteria should be used to interpret a screening ECG because the ECG is subject to variable interpretation.[61]

Laboratory and other ancillary studies
Studies do not support the use of routine laboratory or other screening tests, such as urinalysis, complete blood count, chemistry profile, lipid profile, ferritin level, or spirometry during the PPE.[100–103] At present, screening for sickle cell trait in NCAA athletes is the only requirement and based on the results of litigation. In light of these recommendations, several investigators have recommended screening for specific conditions, especially in specific athletic populations.

Athletes with sickle cell trait often participate in all activities. These athletes may experience exertional sickling in association with other risk factors (elevation, dehydration, and/or acute illness). In 2010, the NCAA implemented a requirement that all incoming athletes must have their sickle cell status determined before participation, although an individual athlete may decline screening.[104] Of note, sickle cell trait is associated with 2% of deaths in NCAA football players.[105]

Because the prevalence of exercise-induced bronchoconstriction (EIB) in athletes has been reported to range from 6% to 12% to nearly 21% in a group of elite athletes, screening for this condition is often recommended.[106–109] Despite this relatively high prevalence, the ability to successfully screen for this condition is difficult. The sensitivity and specificity of testing for EIB are inadequate for an effective medical screening tool.

Patients with a known history of asthma may require additional evaluation and treatment. These individuals should be risk stratified based on their symptoms: mild intermittent, mild persistent, moderate, or severe. In addition, specific asthma triggers should be identified if possible. Athletes with well-controlled asthma who are asymptomatic at rest and with exertion can be safely cleared after a PPE.[110] If the athlete has not been diagnosed with asthma and exhibits symptoms suggestive of the diagnosis, pulmonary function testing should be considered with consideration for testing preexercise and postexercise. Athletes who are actively wheezing or recovering from an asthma exacerbation should be restricted from participation until symptoms have stabilized. Athletes with asthma should be required to have a rescue inhaler immediately available.

Because of the impact of a sports-related concussion history and understanding that many athletes will not realize previously experienced symptoms may be related to a sports-related concussion, a detailed concussion history is important.[111–113] This history may identify athletes who are high risk for recurrent concussive injury and provides an opportunity for the health care provider to educate the athlete. The history should include specific questions as to previous symptoms of a concussion, length of recovery, and number of perceived concussive injuries. The history should also include information about all previous head, face, or cervical spine injuries. Although no published controlled studies at the present time provide an evidence-based decision regarding baseline neuropsychological assessment, the expert consensus group from the 5th International Conference on Concussion in Sport noted that baseline neuropsychological assessment and testing have clinical value and contribute to the evaluation of suspected sports-related concussion.[114] At this time, baseline or preseason neuropsychological testing is not thought to be required.

The PPE is only 1 aspect of an overall program of risk assessment for athletic participation. In addition to the PPE, physicians should consider exploring other aspects of sports participation to assist athletes in reducing the risk of injury. Practice patterns, rules, equipment, or other factors may have a greater effect on decreasing the mortality and morbidity associated with athletic participation. A marked decrease in cervical spine injuries occurred following the rule change in football banning both deliberate "spearing" and the use of the top of the helmet as the initial point of contact in making a tackle.[115]

Finally, the PPE is an opportunity to review other areas of potential harm to the athlete. Distracted driving, seatbelts, substance use, suicide, and domestic violence are some specific areas of concern. Cardiovascular deaths in young athletes in the United States each year are much less frequent than other causes of death in the same age group.[65] Motor vehicle accidents are a leading cause of death in the young age group and are more common than such events during sports; many are linked to alcohol consumption or cellular phone distraction and therefore are largely preventable.[65]

DETERMINATION OF CLEARANCE

Occasionally, an abnormality or condition is found that may limit an athlete's participation or predispose him or her to further injury. In these cases, the examining physician should review the following questions as the overall question of participation is being debated[37]:

1. Does the problem place the athlete at increased risk for injury?
2. Is another participant at risk for injury because of the problem?
3. Can the athlete safely participate with treatment (ie, medication, rehabilitation, bracing, or padding)?
4. Can limited participation be allowed while treatment is being completed?
5. If clearance is denied only for certain sports or sport categories, in what activities can the athlete safely participate?

A specific risk-analysis providing the physician with further guidance in answering the above questions has not been developed. Furthermore, the specific threshold used in the decision is dependent on numerous factors, including the specific sport, desires of the athlete and parent, and available equipment.

The determination of clearance to participate in a particular sport should be individualized. Guidelines such as the recommendations by the American Academy of Pediatrics and the 2015 *Eligibility and Disqualification Recommendations for Competitive Athletes with Cardiovascular Abnormalities: A Scientific Statement from the American Heart Association and American College of Cardiology* should be considered.[116,117] Participation recommendations are individualized and based on the specific diagnosis, although multiple factors, such as the classification of the sport and the specific health status of the athlete, affect the decision. Whether these specific guidelines for clearance effectively limit participation of athletes at risk for further injury without limiting participation for athletes with minimal or no risk is unclear and has yet to be studied. Furthermore, the effect of inappropriately excluding the individual with minimal or no risk of athletic associated injury or death is unclear.

ADDITIONAL CONSIDERATIONS

Although current research demonstrates that the PPE has no effect on the overall morbidities and mortalities in athletes, other objectives may be fulfilled by these examinations. The determination of general health, the counseling on health-related issues, and the assessment of fitness level for specific sports are several other objectives often identified as being fulfilled during the PPE. Furthermore, no harmful effects of these examinations have been reported. The PPE has also become institutionalized in the athletic and sports medicine community. As such, physicians should base their PPE on the best available evidence using the standard PPE form, such as the one recommended by Bernhardt and Roberts.[37]

In general, the current recommended PPE fails to meet many of its intended objectives, including the detection of conditions that may predispose to injury or conditions that may be life threatening or disabling. This ineffectiveness has been studied by several investigators. Glover and Maron[118] found that the preparticipation athletic screening for cardiovascular disease in US high schools may be inadequate, is implemented by a variety of health care providers with varying levels of expertise, and may be severely limited in its power to detect potentially lethal cardiovascular abnormalities. Gomez and colleagues[119] found that 17.2% of high schools used PPE forms with all the elements of the cardiac history recommended by the consensus panel, and the PPE varies among states. Although an effective screening tool has yet to developed, many authorities think the preparticipation screening process used by many US colleges and universities appear to have limited potential to detect cardiovascular abnormalities capable of causing sudden death in competitive student athletes based on the finding that untested guidelines were not being met.[120]

These observations may represent an impetus for change and improvement in the preparticipation screening process for high school athletes. Unfortunately, the standardized evaluation that has been recommended has not been shown to be better than the reported inadequate forms used by some states or even to no preparticipation screening. Even when completed by physicians with sports medicine training and experience, an early study found that more than one-third of athletes reported having had a bad-quality preparticipation sports examination.[121] According to these athletes, medical history taking was poor, and physical examination was restricted to blood pressure measurement and/or chest listening and not targeted enough to past athletic injuries. No recent information regarding the perceived quality of these evaluations is present.

DISCLOSURE

The authors have nothing to disclose.

REFERENCES

1. Runyan DK. The pre-participation examination of the young athlete. Clin Pediatr 1983;22:674–9.
2. Strong WB, Steed D. Cardiovascular evaluation of the young athlete. Prim Care 1984;11:61–75.
3. Rowland TW. Preparticipation sports examination of the child and adolescent athlete: changing views of an old ritual. Pediatrician 1986;13:3–9.
4. Kibler WB, Chandler TJ, Uhl T, et al. A musculoskeletal approach to the preparticipation physical examination. Am J Sports Med 1989;17:525–31.
5. McKeag DB. Preparticipation screening of the potential athlete. Clin Sports Med 1989;8:373–97.
6. Fields KB, Delaney M. Focusing the preparticipation sports examination. J Fam Pract 1990;30:304–12.
7. Garrick JG. Orthopedic preparticipation screening examination. Ped Clin North Am 1990;37:1047–56.
8. Tanji JL. The preparticipation physical examination for sports. Am Fam Physician 1990;42:397–402.
9. Ball RM. The sports preparticipation evaluation. N Engl J Med 1991;88:629–33.
10. Smith DM, Lombardo JA, Robinson JB. The preparticipation evaluation. Prim Care 1991;18:777–807.
11. Dyment PG. The orthopedic component of the preparticipation examination. Pediatr Ann 1992;21:159–62.
12. Henderson JM. The preparticipation screening evaluation. J MAG 1992;81:277–82.
13. Hoekelman RA. The preparticipation sports physical examination (editorial). Pediatr Ann 1992;21:145–6.
14. Overbaugh KA, Allen JG. The adolescent athlete. Part I: preseason preparation and examination. J Pediatr Health Care 1994;8:146–51.
15. Strong WB. Preparticipation physical examination. Arch Pediatr Adolesc Med 1994;1994:99–100.
16. Hergenroeder AC. The preparticipation sports examination. Ped Clin North Am 1997;44:1525–40.
17. Bratton RL. Preparticipation screening of children for sports. Sports Med 1997;24:300–7.
18. Cantwell JD. Preparticipation physical evaluation: getting to the heart of the matter. Med Sci Sports Exerc 1998;10(suppl):S341–4.
19. Clinkenbeard D, Wright P. The preparticipation physical examination and its current status in Oklahoma. J Okla State Med Assoc 1998;91:155–61.
20. Myers A, Sickles T. Preparticipation sports examination. Prim Care Clin Off Pract 1998;25:225–36.
21. Metzl JD. The adolescent preparticipation physical examination: is it helpful? Clin Sports Med 2000;19.

22. Lyznicki JM, Nielsen NH, Schneider JF. Cardiovascular screening of student athletes. Am Fam Physician 2000;62:765–84.
23. McKeag DB, Sallis RE. Factors at play in the athletic preparticipation examination. Am Fam Physician 2000;61.
24. Stickler GB. Are yearly physical examinations in adolescents necessary? J Am Board Fam Pract 2000;13:172–7.
25. Carek PJ, Hunter MH. The preparticipation physical examination for athletes: a critical review of current recommendations. J Med Leban 2001;49:292–7.
26. Lombardo JA, Badolato SK. The preparticipation physical examination. Clin Cornerstone 2001;3:10–25.
27. Carek PJ, Mainous AG. A thorough yet efficient exam identifies most problems in school athletes. J Fam Pract 2003;52:127–34.
28. Seto CK. Preparticipation cardiovascular screening. Clin Sports Med 2003;22: 23–35.
29. Armsey TD, Hosey RG. Medical aspects of sports: epidemiology of injuries, preparticipation physical examination, and drugs in sports. Clin Sports Med 2004; 23:255–79.
30. Wingfield K, Matheson GO, Meeuwisse WH. Preparticipation evaluation: an evidence-based review. Clin J Sport Med 2004;14:109–22.
31. Seto CK. The preparticipation physical examination: an update. Clin Sports Med 2011;30:491–501.
32. Roberts WO, Löllgen H, Matheson GO, et al. Advancing the preparticipation physical evaluation (PPE): an ACSM and FIMS joint consensus statement. Curr Sports Med Rep 2014;13(6):395–401.
33. Mirabelli MH, Devine MJ, Singh J, et al. The preparticipation sports evaluation. Am Fam Physician 2015;92(5):371–6.
34. Kris PK, Clyne A, Ford SR. Preparticipation physical exams: the Rhode Island Experience, a call for standardization. R I Med J 2016;99(10):18–22.
35. Drezner JA, O'Connor FG, Harmon KG, et al. AMSSM position statement on cardiovascular preparticipation screening for athletes: current evidence, knowledge gaps, recommendations and future directions. Br J Sports Med 2017; 51:153–67.
36. Lehman PJ, Carl RL. The preparticipation physical evaluation. Pediatr Ann 2017; 46(3):e85–92.
37. Bernhardt DT, Roberts WO, editors. Preparticipation physical evaluation. 4th Edition. Elk Grove Village (IL): American Academy of Pediatrics; 2010.
38. Maron BJ, Thompson PD, Ackerman MJ, et al. Recommendations and considerations related to preparticipation screening for cardiovascular abnormalities in competitive athletes: 2007 update: a scientific statement from the American Heart Association Council on Nutrition, Physical Activity, and Metabolism: endorsed by the American College of Cardiology Foundation. Circulation 2007;115(12). 1643–455.
39. Maron BJ, Levine BD, Washington RL, et al. Eligibility and disqualification recommendations for competitive athletes with cardiovascular abnormalities: task force 2: preparticipation screening for cardiovascular disease in competitive athletes: a scientific statement from the American Heart Association and American College of Cardiology. J Am Coll Cardiol 2015;66(21):2356–61.
40. Mont L, Pelliccia A, Sharma S, et al. Pre-participation cardiovascular evaluation for athletic participants to prevent sudden death: position paper from the EHRA and the EACPR, branches of the ESC. Endorsed by APHRS, HRS, and SOLAECE. Eur J Prev Cardiol 2017;24(1):41–69.

41. MacAuley D. Does the preseason screening for cardiac disease really work?: the British perspective. Med Sci Sports Exerc 1998;30:S345–50.
42. Batt ME, Jacques R, Stone M. Preparticipation examination (screening): practical issues as determined by sport. Clin J Sport Med 2004;14:178–82.
43. Lollgen H, Leyk D, Hansel J. The preparticipation examination for leisure time physical activity. Dtsch Arztebl Int 2010;107:742–9.
44. Jenoure PJ. The preparticipation physical examination in Europe: all around the pre-participation examination. European Federation of Sports Medicine Federations. Available at: www.efsma.net. Accessed April 15, 2019.
45. Krowchuk DP, Krowchuk HV, Hunter M, et al. Parents' knowledge of the purposes and content of preparticipation physical examinations. Arch Pediatr Adolesc Med 1995;149:653–7.
46. Carek PJ, Futrell MA. Athlete's view of the preparticipation physical examination: attitudes toward certain health screening questions. Arch Fam Med 1999;8: 307–12.
47. Goldberg B, Saranti A, Witman P, et al. Pre-participation sports assessment: an objective evaluation. Pediatrics 1980;66(5):736–45.
48. Linder CW, DuRant RH, Seklecki RM, et al. Preparticipation health screening of young athletes: results of 1268 examinations. Am J Sports Med 1981;9(3): 187–93.
49. Tennant FS Jr, Sorenson K, Day CM. Benefits of preparticipation sports examinations. J Fam Pract 1981;13(2):287–8.
50. Thompson TR, Andrish JT, Bergfield JA. A prospective study of preparticipation sports examinations of 2670 young athletes: method and results. Cleve Clin Q 1982;49(4):225–33.
51. DuRant RH, Pendergrast RA, Seymore C, et al. Findings from the preparticipation athletic examination and athletic injuries. Am J Dis Child 1992;146:85–91.
52. Risser WL, Hoffman HM, Bellah GG Jr. Frequency of preparticipation sports examinations in secondary school athletes: are the University Interscholastic League guidelines appropriate? Tex Med 1985;81(7):35–9.
53. Magnes SA, Henderson JM, Hunter SC. What limits sports participation: experience with 10,540 athletes. Phys Sportsmed 1992;20:143–60.
54. Rifat SF, Ruffin MT, Gorenflo DW. Disqualifying criteria in preparticipation sports evaluation. J Fam Pract 1995;41:42–50.
55. Lively MW. Preparticipation physical examination: a collegiate experience. Clin J Sports Med 1999;9(1):38.
56. Mayer F, Bonaventura K, Cassel M, et al. Medical results of preparticipation examination in adolescent athletes. Br J Sports Med 2012;46(7):524–30.
57. Smith DM, Kovan JR, Rich BSE, et al. Preparticipation physical evaluation. 2nd edition. Minneapolis (MN): McGraw-Hill Co; 1997. p. 1–46.
58. American Medical Association Board of Trustees, Group on Science and Technology. Athletic participation examinations for adolescents. Arch Pediatr Adolesc Med 1994;148:93–8.
59. Roberts WO, Stovitz S. Incidence of sudden cardiac death in Minnesota high school athletes 1993Y2012 screened with a standardized preparticipation evaluation. J Am Coll Cardiol 2013;62:1298–301.
60. Drezner JA, Rao AL, Heistand J, et al. Effectiveness of emergency response planning for sudden cardiac arrest in United States high schools with automated external defibrillators. Circulation 2009;120:518–25.
61. Drezner JA, Sharma A, Baggish A, et al. International criteria for electrocardiographic interpretation in athletes. Br J Sports Med 2017;1:1–28.

62. Asif IM, Harmon KG. Incidence and etiology of sudden cardiac death: new up-dates for athletic departments. Sports Health 2017;9(3):268–79.
63. Harmon KG, Drezner JA, Wilson MG, et al. Incidence of sudden cardiac death in athletes: a state-of-the art review. Br J Sports Med 2014;48:1185–92.
64. Mechelen W, Twisk J, Molendijk A, et al. Subject-related risk factors for sports injuries: a 1-yr prospective study in young adults. Med Sci Sports Exerc 1996; 28:1171–9.
65. Maron BJ, Friedman RA, Kligfield P, et al. Assessment of the 12-lead ECG as a screening test for detection of cardiovascular disease in healthy general popu-lations of young people (12-25 years of age). J Am Coll Cardiol 2014;64(14): 1479–514.
66. Rumbell JS, Lebrun CM. Preparticipation physical examination: selected issues for the female athlete. Clin J Sport Med 2004;14:153–60.
67. De Souza MJ, Nattiv A, Joy E, et al. 2014 female athlete triad coalition consensus statement on treatment and return to play of the female athlete triad: 1st International Conference held in San Francisco, California, May 2012 and 2nd International Conference held in Indianapolis, Indiana, May 2013. Br J Sports Med 2014;48(4):289.
68. Carek PJ, Futrell MA, Hueston WJ. The preparticipation physical examination history: who has the correct answer? Clin J Sports Med 1999;9:124–8.
69. Huston TP, Puffer JC, Rodney WM. The athletic heart syndrome. N Engl J Med 1985;313:24–32.
70. Crawford MH, O'Rourke RA. The athlete's heart. Adv Intern Med 1979;24: 311–29.
71. Gomez JE, Landry GL, Bernhardt DT. Critical evaluation of the 2-minute orthope-dic screening examination. Am J Dis Child 1993;147:1109–13.
72. Abbott HG, Kress JB. Preconditioning in the prevention of knee injuries. Arch Phys Med Rehabil 1969;50:326–33.
73. Jackson DW, Jarrett H, Bailey D, et al. Injury prediction in the young athlete: a preliminary report. Am J Sports Med 1978;6:6–14.
74. Nicholas JA. Injuries in knee ligaments: relationship to looseness and tightness in football players. JAMA 1970;212:2236–9.
75. Willems TM, Witvrouw E, Delbaere K, et al. Intrinsic risk factors for inversion ankle sprains in male subjects. Am J Sports Med 2005;33:415–23.
76. Meeuwisse WH, Fowler PJ. Frequency and predictability of sports injuries in intercollegiate athletes. Can J Sports Sci 1988;13:35–42.
77. Garrick JG. Preparticipation orthopedic screening evaluation. Clin J Sport Med 2004;14:123–6.
78. Thacker SB, Gilchrist J, Stroup DF, et al. The impact of stretching on sports injury risk: a systematic review of the literature. Med Sci Sports Exerc 2004; 36(3):371–8.
79. Smith J, Laskowski E. The preparticipation physical examination: Mayo Clinic experience with 2,739 examinations. Mayo Clin Proc 1998;73:419–29.
80. Fitzgibbons RJ, Giobbie-Hurder A, Gibbs JO, et al. Watchful waiting vs repair of inguinal hernia in minimally symptomatic men. JAMA 2006;295(3):285–92.
81. Lewis JF, Maron BJ, Diggs JA, et al. Preparticipation echocardiographic screening for cardiovascular disease in a large, predominately black population of collegiate athletes. Am Coll Cardiol 1989;64(16):1029–33.
82. Maron BJ, Klues HG. Surviving competitive athletes with hypertrophic cardiomy-opathy. Am J Card 1994;73(15):1098–104.

83. Fuller CM, McNulty CM, Spring DA, et al. Prospective screening of 5,615 high school athletes for risk of sudden death. Med Sci Sports Exerc 1997;29(9): 1131–8.
84. Fuller CM. Cost effectiveness of analysis of high school athletes for risks of sudden death. Med Sci Sports Exerc 2000;32:887–90.
85. Pelliccia A, Maron BJ, Culasso F, et al. Clinical significance of abnormal electrocardiographic patterns in trained athletes. Circulation 2000;102(3):278–84.
86. Corrado D, Basso C, Pavei A, et al. Trends in sudden cardiovascular death in young competitive athletes after implementation of a preparticipation screening program. JAMA 2006;291:1593–601.
87. Steinvil A, Chundadze T, Zeltser D, et al. Mandatory electrocardiographic screening of athletes to reduce their risk for sudden death proven fact or wishful thinking? J Am Coll Cardiol 2011;57:1291–6.
88. Yanai O, Phillips ED, Hiss J. Sudden cardiac death during sport and recreational activities in Israel. J Clin Forensic Med 2000;7:88–91.
89. Ma JZ, Dai J, Sun B, et al. Cardiovascular preparticipation screening of young competitive athletes for prevention of sudden death in China. J Sci Med Sport 2007;10:227–33.
90. Beckerman J, Wang P, Hlatky M. Cardiovascular screening of athletes. Clin J Sports Med 2004;14:127–33.
91. Malhotra A, Dhutia H, Finocchiaro G, et al. Outcomes of cardiac screening in adolescent soccer players. N Engl J Med 2018;379:524–34.
92. Maron BJ, Haas TS, Ahluwalia A, et al. Incidence of cardiovascular sudden deaths in Minnesota high school athletes. Heart Rhythm 2013;10:374–7.
93. Harmon KG, Asif IM, Klossner D, et al. Incidence of sudden cardiac death in National Collegiate Athletic Association athletes. Circulation 2011;123:1594–600.
94. Brugada P, Brugada J. Right bundle branch block, persistent ST segment elevation and sudden cardiac death: a distinct clinical and electrocardiographic syndrome. A multicenter report. J Am Coll Cardiol 1992;20:1391–6.
95. Maron BJ, Haas TS, Doerer JJ, et al. Comparison of U.S. and Italian experiences with sudden cardiac deaths in young competitive athletes and implications for preparticipation screening strategies. Am J Cardiol 2009;104:276–80.
96. Harmon KG, Asif IM, Maleszewski JJ, et al. Incidence, cause, and comparative frequency of sudden cardiac death in National Collegiate Athletic Association Athletes: a decade in review. Circulation 2015;132(1):10–9.
97. Roberts WO, Asplund CA, O'Connor FG, et al. Cardiac preparticipation screening for the young athlete: why the routine use of ECG is not necessary. J Electrocardiol 2015;48:311–5.
98. Asplund CA, O'Connor. The evidence against cardiac screening using electrocardiogram in athletes. Curr Sports Med Rep 2016;15(2):81–5.
99. Asif IM, Drezner JA. Cardiovascular screening in young athletes: evidence for the electrocardiogram. Curr Sports Med Rep 2016;15(2):76–80.
100. Dodge WF WF, West EF, Smith, et al. Proteinuria and hematuria in schoolchildren: Epidemiology and early natural history. J Pediatr 1976;88(2):327–47.
101. Peggs JF, Reinhardt RW, O'Brien JM. Proteinuria in adolescent sports physical examinations. J Fam Pract 1986;22(1):80–1.
102. Rupp NT, Brudno DS, Guill MF. The value of screening for risk of exercise-induced asthma in high school athletes. Ann Allergy 1993;70(4):339–42.
103. Feinstein RA, La Russa J, Wang-Dohlman A, et al. Screening adolescent athletes for exercise-induced asthma. Clin J Sports Med 1996;6(2):119–23.

104. Klossner D, National Collegiate Athletic Association. 2018-19 NCAA sports medicine handbook. Available at: http://www.ncaapublications.com/productdownloads/D119.pdf. Accessed April 10, 2019.
105. Harmon KG, Drezner JA, Klossner D, et al. Sickle cell trait associated with a RR of death of 37 times in National Collegiate Athletic Association football athletes: a database with 2 million athlete-years as the denominator. Br J Sports Med 2012;46(5):325–30.
106. Corrigan B, Kazlauskas R. Medication use in athletes selected for doping control at the Sydney Olympics (2000). Clin J Sport Med 2003;13:33–40.
107. Randolph C, Randolph M, Fraser B. Exercise-induced asthma in school children. J Allergy Clin Immunol 1991;87:341.
108. Kawabori I, Pierson WE, Conquest LL, et al. Incidence of exercise-induced asthma in children. J Allergy Clin Immunol 1976;58:447–55.
109. Rupp NT, Guill MF, Brudno DS. Unrecognized exercise-induced bronchospasm in adolescent athletes. Am J Dis Child 1992;146:941–4.
110. Hong G, Mahamitra N. Medical screening of the athlete: how does asthma fit in? Clin Rev Allergy Immunol 2005;29(2):97–111.
111. Delaney J, Lacroix V, Leclerc S, et al. Canadian football league season. Clin J Sport Med 1997;2000:9–14.
112. Delaney JS, Lacroix VJ, LeclercS, et al. Concussions among university football and soccer players. Clin J Sport Med 2002;12:331–8.
113. McCrory P. Preparticipation assessment for head injury. Clin J Sport Med 2004; 14:139–44.
114. McCrory P, Meeuwisse W, Dvorak J, et al. Consensus statement on concussion in sport–the 5th International Conference on concussion in sport held in Berlin, October 2016. Br J Sports Med 2018;51:838–47.
115. Torg JS, Vegso JJ, Sennett B, et al. The National Football Head and Neck Injury Registry: 14-year report on cervical quadriplegia, 1971 through 1984. JAMA 1985;254(24):3439–43.
116. Rice SG. Medical conditions affecting sports participation. Pediatrics 2008; 121(4):841–8.
117. Maron BJ, Zipes DP, Kovacs RJ. Eligibility and disqualification recommendations for competitive athletes with cardiovascular abnormalities: preamble, principles, and general considerations: a scientific statement from the American Heart Association and American College of Cardiology. J Am Coll Cardiol 2015;66(21):2343–9.
118. Glover DW, Maron BJ. Profile of preparticipation cardiovascular screening for high school athletes. JAMA 1998;279:1817–9.
119. Gomez JE, Lantry BR, Saathoff KN. Current use of adequate preparticipation history forms for heart disease screening of high school athletes. Arch Pediatr Adolesc Med 1999;153:723–6.
120. Pfister GC, Puffer JC, Maron BJ. Preparticipation cardiovascular screening for US collegiate student-athletes. JAMA 2000;283:1597–9.
121. Laure P. High-level athlete's impressions of their preparticipation sports examination. J Sports Med Phys Fitness 1996;36:291–2.
122. DuRant R, Seymore C, Linder CW, et al. The preparticipation examination of athletes: Comparison of single and multiple examiners. Am J Dis Child 1985;139:657–61.

Detection and Management of Heart Disease in Athletes

David M. Siebert, MD*, Jonathan A. Drezner, MD

KEYWORDS

- Athlete • Cardiovascular disease • Electrocardiogram • Sudden cardiac arrest
- Preparticipation physical evaluation (PPE) • Athlete's heart • International Criteria
- Sports cardiology

KEY POINTS

- Cardiovascular disease encompasses a heterogeneous group of primary structural and electrical disorders in young athletes and chiefly coronary artery disease in older athletes.
- Sudden cardiac arrest may be the initial presentation of disease in both groups and occurs more frequently in young athletes than historical estimates would indicate.
- The traditional preparticipation evaluation is limited in its ability to detect underlying cardiovascular disease in young athletes.
- The 12-lead electrocardiogram is a more sensitive tool than the traditional preparticipation evaluation for raising suspicion of occult conditions, but its optimal implementation into screening programs remains an area of intense research and debate.
- Contemporary risk stratification and treatment guidelines may allow for safe return to sport on a case-by-case basis, with specialist consultation.

INTRODUCTION

Cardiovascular disease (CVD) remains the leading cause of death in the United States.[1] Although this statistic is perhaps not surprising in older patients with classic risk factors, such as hypertension or dyslipidemia, sudden cardiac arrest (SCA) also accounts for the majority of exercise-related deaths in young athletes.[2,3] The burden of CVD, in addition to widespread agreement that physical activity promotes and maintains cardiovascular health,[4,5] uniquely places the primary care clinician in a critical role for screening, evaluation, and management of a variety of patients and conditions to foster cardiovascular health.

Given the increasing emphasis on the benefits of sports and exercise in all ages and walks of life, the responsibilities of the primary care provider may include

Department of Family Medicine, UW Medicine Center for Sports Cardiology, University of Washington, 3800 Montlake Boulevard NE, Seattle, WA 98195, USA
* Corresponding author.
E-mail address: siebert@uw.edu

Prim Care Clin Office Pract 47 (2020) 19–35
https://doi.org/10.1016/j.pop.2019.11.001
0095-4543/20/© 2019 Elsevier Inc. All rights reserved.
primarycare.theclinics.com

- Conducting preparticipation cardiovascular screening in pediatric athletes
- Performing the initial evaluation and management of suspected CVD in the young athlete
- Managing risk reduction in the active or newly active adult with or without diagnosed CVD

From elite athletes to weekend warriors, primary care providers have a unique opportunity to help patients of all ages engage in safe exercise and maintain an active lifestyle. This article provides a contemporary review of the epidemiology, detection, and management of CVD in athletes.

ETIOLOGY OF SUDDEN CARDIAC ARREST AND DEATH IN YOUNG COMPETITIVE ATHLETES
Overview

The diseases and conditions associated with SCA and sudden cardiac death (SCD) in the young athlete (<35 years old) comprise a heterogeneous group of congenital or acquired structural and electrical disorders. These include primary cardiomyopathies, coronary artery anomalies, channelopathies, valvular disorders, and diseases of ventricular preexcitation, among others.[2,3,6,7] Hypertrophic cardiomyopathy (HCM) is classically considered the most frequent cause of SCD in athletes, having been identified as the underlying etiology in as many as 36% of cases, a rate more than twice as frequent as the second leading cause of anomalous coronary arteries (17%).[3] More recent research, however, has identified more than 15 different etiologies of SCA/SCD in United States athletes, with HCM (16.2%), coronary artery anomalies (13.7%), and idiopathic left ventricular hypertrophy (11.1%), representing relatively smaller proportions of a diverse group of conditions[6] (Table 1). HCM was identified more frequently as the underlying etiology in African American athletes compared with white athletes (P<.05).[6] Autopsy-negative sudden unexplained death (AN-SUD), implying primary electrical disease that could not be identified postmortem, also is a common finding in SCD cases.[2] AN-SUD has been found to be the leading cause of SCA/SCD in some international studies,[8,9] whereas cardiomyopathies, such as HCM, are the leading causes in others.[10,11] Variable study populations, differing postmortem examination criteria, and lack of a standardized methodology of case identification from region to region or country to country may account for discrepancies between studies.

Certain conditions merit special attention as the most common causes of SCA/SCD that may be encountered in primary care practices.

Hypertrophic Cardiomyopathy

HCM is a condition characterized by increased left ventricular wall thickness that is usually asymmetric and involves the interventricular septum. HCM affects as many as 1 in 500 people worldwide, with more than 1400 different genetic mutations described. Abnormal wall thickness combined with systolic anterior motion of the mitral valve can lead to left ventricular outflow tract obstruction and potential symptoms of exertional dyspnea, chest pain, or syncope, but a majority of cases in young athletes are asymptomatic prior to the sentinel event of SCA. SCA stems from a disorganized myocardial architecture and arrhythmogenic foci of interstitial fibrosis.[12]

A resting 12-lead electrocardiogram (ECG) is abnormal in as many as 96% of cases of HCM.[13] Classic ECG findings suggestive of HCM include T-wave inversions (TWIs) in the lateral or inferolateral leads with concurrent ST-segment depressions (Fig. 1). These ECG findings are highly suggestive of cardiomyopathy and must not be

Table 1
Etiology of Sudden Cardiac Arrest and Death in Competitive Athletes: July 1, 2014, to June 30, 2016 (n = 117[a])

	Sudden Cardiac Arrest (n = 34), N (%)	Sudden Cardiac Death (n = 83), N (%)	Total, N (%)
HCM	4 (11.8)	15 (18.1)	19 (16.2)
Coronary artery anomalies	3 (8.8)	13 (15.7)	16 (13.7)
Anomalous origin LCA	—	10	—
Agenesis of LCA ostium	—	1	—
Anomalous RCA with aberrant takeoff and hypoplasia	—	1	—
Myocardial bridging	—	1	—
Idiopathic left ventricular hypertrophy/possible cardiomyopathy	—	13 (15.7)	13 (11.1)
AN-SUD	—	8 (9.6)	8 (6.8)
WPW	6 (17.6)	2 (2.4)	8 (6.8)
LQTS	4 (11.8)	3 (3.6)	7 (6.0)
Arrhythmogenic cardiomyopathy	2 (5.9)	4 (4.8)	6 (5.1)
Dilated cardiomyopathy	2 (5.9)	4 (4.8)	6 (5.1)
Aortic dissection/rupture	0 (0)	5 (6.0)	5 (4.3)
Associated bicuspid aortic valve	—	2	—
Associated Marfan syndrome	—	1	—
Myocarditis	2 (5.9)	3 (3.6)	5 (4.3)
Complications of a congenital heart defect	1 (2.9)	3 (3.6)	4 (3.4)
Ebstein anomaly	—	1	—
Left ventricular hypertrophy associated with congenital aortic stenosis	—	1	—
Transposition of the great arteries	—	1	—
Tetralogy of Fallot	1	—	—
Coronary atherosclerosis	2 (5.9)	2 (2.4)	4 (3.4)
Valvular disorder	1 (2.9)	2 (2.4)	3 (2.6)
Commotio cordis	3 (8.8)	0 (0)	3 (2.6)
Catecholaminergic polymorphic ventricular tachycardia	2 (5.9)	0 (0)	2 (1.7)
Hypertensive heart disease	0(0)	2 (2.4)	2 (1.7)
Restrictive cardiomyopathy	1 (2.9)	0 (0)	1 (0.9)
Left ventricular noncompaction	0 (0)	1 (1.2)	1 (0.9)
Fibromuscular dysplasia of the sinoatrial nodal artery	0 (0)	1 (1.2)	1 (0.9)
Paroxysmal atrial tachycardia	0 (0)	1 (1.2)	1 (0.9)
Right atrial myxoma	0 (0)	1 (1.2)	1 (0.9)
Pericarditis	1 (2.9)	0 (0)	1 (0.9)

[a] One hundred seventeen (65.4%) cases had a reported or adjudicated diagnosis.

From Peterson DF, Siebert DM, Kucera KL, et al. Etiology of sudden cardiac arrest and death in US competitive athletes: a 2-year prospective surveillance study. Clin J Sport Med. 2018;(Apr 9):6; with permission.

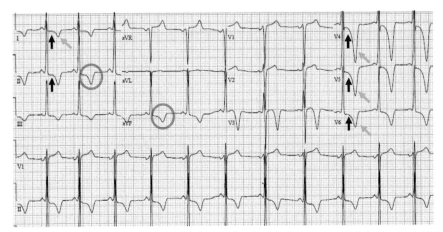

Fig. 1. Abnormal ECG findings, notably lateral lead TWIs (*blue arrows*), inferior lead TWIs (*red circles*), and lateral lead ST segment depressions (*black arrows*), that are suggestive of HCM and thus require further investigation.

discounted without appropriate follow-up testing and consultation.[14] Conversely, training-related left ventricular hypertrophy from athlete's heart does not exhibit lateral TWIs, and voltage criteria for left ventricular hypertrophy are a common finding in athletes (**Fig. 2**). Isolated left ventricular hypertrophy on ECG, when found in isolation and without other ECG abnormalities, symptoms, or family history concerns, is not a distinguishing finding for pathology and is considered a normal finding in trained athletes.[14]

Transthoracic echocardiogram (TTE) may be sufficient to make an initial HCM diagnosis, although a negative TTE does not exclude HCM involving the anterolateral wall or apex, especially when clinical suspicion is high or when markedly abnormal ECG findings are identified (see **Fig. 1**). In this case, cardiac magnetic resonance imaging (MRI) should be a routine test in the evaluation of athletes with lateral or inferolateral

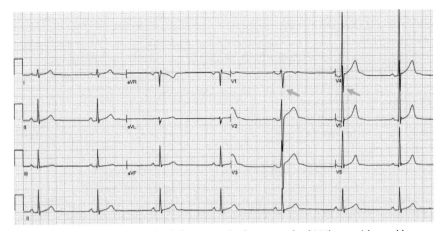

Fig. 2. Isolated voltage criteria for left ventricular hypertrophy (LVH), as evidenced by a sum of the S wave in V1 and R wave in V5 of greater than 35 mm (*blue arrows*). Note the lack of TWIs or ST depressions. LVH in isolation is considered a normal variant in trained athletes.

TWIs to exclude apical HCM, arrhythmogenic cardiomyopathy with left ventricular involvement, or nonischemic left ventricular scar.[14]

If diagnosed, management of HCM should include close consultation with a cardiologist, preferably one with experience in cardiomyopathy or sports cardiology. The athlete should be restricted from strenuous exercise and competitive sports until further work-up can be completed and the optimal care plan determined. Additional risk stratification includes assessment with exercise stress testing and 24-hour ambulatory ECG monitoring. Family screening and genetic testing also should be considered.[12] Based on current guidelines by the American Heart Association (AHA) and the American College of Cardiology (ACC), probable or unequivocal clinical expression of any degree or variety of HCM is considered a contraindication to all but low-intensity competitive sports,[15] and morbidity-reducing treatment should be pursued via specialist consultation.[16] Treatment may include pharmacologic management, implantable cardioverter-defibrillator (ICD) placement, or other procedural interventions, such as surgical myomectomy.[12] Regular specialist follow-up also can inform individual exercise regimens for fitness purposes on a case-by-case basis.[12,16]

Anomalous Coronary Arteries

Coronary artery anomalies are another leading cause of SCA/SCD in athletes. Anomalies include the left coronary artery (LCA) arising from the right sinus of Valsalva or the right coronary artery (RCA) arising from the left sinus of Valsalva. Studies suggest that fewer than 50% of athletes with SCA from an anomalous coronary artery had preexisting warning symptoms of their condition, such as exertional chest pain or syncope.[17]

Coronary artery anomalies appear to precipitate SCA/SCD as a consequence of ischemic changes arising from abnormal artery positioning or formation. For example, an anomalous LCA may be compressed by its intramural course within the wall of the aorta or during exercise as it travels between the aorta and pulmonary arteries, leading to repeat bouts of transient ischemia. These bouts may promote myocardial fibrosis, which may predispose to ventricular arrhythmias.[17]

Anomalous coronary arteries are among the more difficult conditions to detect in their preclinical state.[18] Resting and stress ECGs are frequently normal.[17,19] A high clinical suspicion must be maintained in the athlete with exertional chest pain or syncope. The coronary arteries can be satisfactorily assessed in more than 90% of athletes with a focused TTE,[20] suggesting that if they cannot be visualized in an athlete with unexplained cardiovascular symptoms, computed tomography (CT) angiography or cardiac MRI should be considered.[17]

The treatment of coronary artery anomalies is surgical. According to the AHA, athletes with an anomalous origin of the RCA may participate in sports after counseling, provided an athlete is asymptomatic with a normal exercise stress test. An anomalous LCA is a higher-risk lesion. Competitive sports participation should be restricted until at least 3 months after surgical correction of the lesion, assuming the athlete is asymptomatic with no evidence of ischemia or arrhythmia demonstrated on exercise stress testing.[21]

Wolff-Parkinson-White

Wolff-Parkinson-White (WPW) is a congenital condition characterized by 1 or more accessory conduction pathways within the heart. Classic ECG findings include a short PR interval and the presence of a delta wave (slurred QRS upstroke), signifying ventricular preexcitation (**Fig. 3**). Many patients with WPW are asymptomatic, whereas others may report symptoms suggesting arrhythmias, such as palpitations.[22] WPW

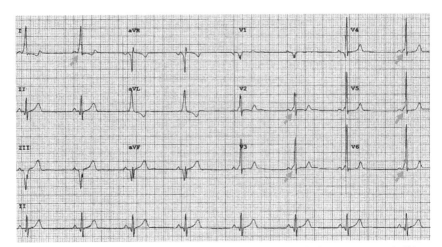

Fig. 3. ECG of a patient with WPW. Note the delta waves with short PR intervals (*blue arrows*). Other WPW findings include large Q waves in lead III and the lack of a Q wave in lead V6.

also is a known cause of SCA/SCD, accounting for 6.8% of all cases in a recent study.[6] SCA/SCD from WPW is thought to arise from the rapid conduction of atrial fibrillation across the accessory pathway, bypassing the rate-controlling atrioventricular node and thus precipitating ventricular fibrillation.[22]

Intermittent ventricular preexcitation, characterized by periodic loss of the delta wave on ECG monitoring, is considered a low-risk pathway that is unlikely to precipitate malignant arrhythmias. Persistent delta waves at rest merit further evaluation, including echocardiography, to assess for structural abnormalities associated with WPW, such as cardiomyopathies or Ebstein anomaly.[22] Exercise stress testing should be used to assess for the abrupt loss of the delta wave with exercise. Athletes who demonstrate persistent delta waves with exercise, or those who participate in moderate-intensity or high-intensity sports, are considered higher risk athletes. Such athletes should be offered consultation with an electrophysiologist for consideration of an electrophysiology study to identify high-risk pathways that may be amenable to ablation.[22,23]

Long QT Syndrome

Long QT syndrome (LQTS) is a genetic ion channelopathy that yields a prolonged QT interval on ECG and may precipitate polymorphic ventricular tachycardia, also known as torsades de pointes.[24] A prolonged QT interval in athletes is defined as a QT interval corrected for heart rate (QTc) using Bazett formula of greater than or equal to 470 ms in male athletes and greater than or equal to 480 ms in female athletes[14] (**Fig. 4**). Importantly, a single ECG with a prolonged QT interval does not equate to a diagnosis of LQTS, which requires confirmation by genetic testing, family screening, and/or paradoxic prolongation of the QT interval during the recovery phase of an exercise stress test. QT prolonging medications or electrolyte abnormalities also should be excluded. Diagnostic criteria have been recommended by the Heart Rhythm Society, the European Heart Rhythm Association, and the Asia Pacific Heart Rhythm Society. These societies recommend a formal diagnosis of LQTS with a Schwartz criteria[25] score of greater than or equal to 3.5, a confirmed LQTS genetic mutation, a QTc of greater

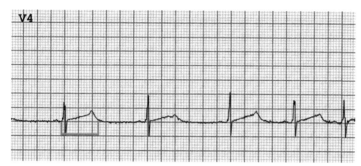

Fig. 4. LQTS. Precordial lead V4 showing a prolonged QT interval (*bracket*).

than or equal to 500 ms, or a QTc between 480 ms and 499 ms with suggestive symptoms, such as unexplained syncope.[26]

Ventricular arrhythmias may be provoked by extreme emotional stress or physical activity, especially swimming, in the setting of LQTS type I and can lead to syncope with seizure-like activity or sudden death.[24] Previously considered a contraindication to competitive sports,[27] recent observational data suggest that athletes with LQTS who undergo optimal medical management and counseling may not be at as high of risk of SCA/SCD as previously postulated.[28–30]

Updated guidelines for the management of LQTS in athletes have been published.[31,32] The medical management of LQTS includes β-blockade in most patients, including those who are asymptomatic, as well as avoiding medications that prolong the QT interval.[26] β-blockers are prohibited in certain competitive sports by the World Anti-Doping Agency.[33] ICD placement should be considered in high-risk athletes, such as those who have survived prior SCA.[26,31] Athletes with ICDs in place may consider returning to competitive sports under contemporary recommendations provided no shocks have been delivered to abort ventricular arrhythmias for at least 3 months. According to the AHA and ACC, however, "the desire of the athlete to continue athletic competition should not represent the primary indication for use of an ICD".[34]

Other Etiologies

SCA/SCD in athletes has been attributed to several other etiologies. Arrhythmogenic right ventricular cardiomyopathy (ARVC) is a condition characterized by the progressive replacement of right ventricular myocardium by arrhythmia-promoting fibrofatty tissue.[35] Responsible for 5% of SCA/SCD in athletes in 1 study,[6] ARVC is suggested by TWIs in the anterior precordial leads (V1-V4) on ECG.[35] Given the difficulty in confirming a diagnosis, formal diagnostic criteria have been proposed.[36,37] Treatment options include β-blockade to prevent SCA and ICD implantation in high-risk patients or those who have survived aborted SCA. In patients with manifestations of ARVC-driven congestive heart failure, appropriate medical therapy should be instituted.[35] The AHA and ACC recommend restriction from competitive sports, except for possibly low-intensity sports, in all patients with possible or confirmed ARVC.[15]

Dilated cardiomyopathy causes approximately 5% of athlete SCA/SCD cases,[6] and the AHA and ACC recommend restricting symptomatic athletes from competition after diagnosis.[15] Other documented SCA/SCD etiologies include aortic dissections or rupture, myocarditis, restrictive cardiomyopathy, catecholaminergic polymorphic ventricular tachycardia, and left ventricular noncompaction cardiomyopathy.[38] SCA/SCD related to commotio cordis, characterized by SCA after direct impact of the chest wall by a blunt object, represents another 3% of cases.[6]

INCIDENCE OF SUDDEN CARDIAC ARREST/SUDDEN CARDIAC DEATH IN THE YOUNG COMPETITIVE ATHLETE

The central goal of an effective screening protocol is to prevent the progression of pre-clinical disease to its clinical state. In the case of CVD in young athletes, SCA can be the initial manifestation of disease,[7,39] making the preclinical detection of pathologic conditions of paramount importance. Epidemiologic data play a crucial role in determining the appropriateness of screening and informing the optimal methods for early detection.

The annual incidence of SCA/SCD in young competitive athletes varies considerably in the published literature. An annual SCD risk of 1:200,000 in high school athletes was proposed as an estimate in the late twentieth century,[40] with rates as low as 1:417,000 also reported.[41] Contemporary research with more extensive methodology, however, has concluded that the risk is substantially higher, with minimum annual risk estimates of 1:50,000 in college athletes and 1:80,000 in high school athletes.[42] The discrepancy between historical and modern incidence estimates has been attributed primarily to research methodology differences, difficulties in identifying cases of SCD, and year-to-year variability.[43] Studies also vary regarding the inclusion of SCA with survival, as opposed to exclusively cases of SCD. Given that exercise-related SCA in competitive athletes carries a modern survival rate of 48%,[44] all major cardiovascular events, including both deaths and survivals, are important to consider when informing optimal screening protocols.

A differential risk among athletes also is present, with some athlete subgroups at considerably higher risk than others. For instance, male and African American athletes are consistently at 3-times to 5-times higher risk of SCA/SCD.[2,3,42,45] Certain sports also show a disproportionately higher risk, with more than 50% of SCA/SCD cases occurring in football and basketball.[6] Most strikingly, male Division I college basketball players have an annual SCD risk of 1:5,000.[2]

THE YOUNG ATHLETE PREPARTICIPATION PHYSICAL EVALUATION

The preparticipation physical evaluation (PPE), or sports physical, is a common encounter in the primary care office. Endorsed by numerous medical societies,[46–48] the chief goals of the PPE, as defined by the American Academy of Pediatrics *Preparticipation Physical Evaluation*, are to

1. Screen for conditions that may be life-threatening or disabling
2. Screen for conditions that may predispose to injury or illness
3. Determine general health
4. Serve as an entry point to the health care system for adolescents
5. Provide an opportunity to initiate discussion on health-related topics[42]

Although exercise has numerous health benefits, exercise can trigger SCA in athletes with an underlying heart disorder.[49] Thus, a crucial and widely practiced component of the PPE is to screen for silent CVD that may place an athlete at risk of SCA/SCD. Traditionally, preparticipation cardiovascular screening includes a standardized symptom and family history questionnaire and a targeted cardiovascular physical examination.[46,47] Positive responses to questions about symptoms, such as exertional chest pain or syncope, the identification of a heart murmur on physical examination, or a significant family history of CVD or sudden death at a young age, constitute a positive screen and require additional investigation to exclude the presence of undiag-nosed CVD.

Despite widespread endorsement and utilization of a screening history and physical examination (H&P), no outcomes data support its ability to reduce cardiovascular morbidity and mortality. In an evidence-based consensus statement, the American Medical Society for Sports Medicine (AMSSM) has recognized the limited utility of the H&P alone to detect occult CVD in young athletes.[48] Limitations of the H&P include its general, nonspecific symptom questions, yielding a high rate of positive responses, and its reliance on accurate and truthful reporting by the athlete.[50] Positive response rates to at least 1 symptom or family history question have been reported in 30% to 36% of high school and college athletes.[51-54]

Although history questionnaires yield a high number of positive responses that can be difficult to clarify, certain H&P clues must never be discounted. A history of exercise-related syncope, specifically collapse during exercise, requires a compre-hensive investigation to rule out a cardiac cause. Additionally, a family history of a car-diovascular disorder or sudden death at a young age (<40 years) is suggestive of a possible heritable cardiovascular condition. Physical stigmata of Marfan syndrome or heart murmurs that suggest left ventricular outflow tract obstruction, such as in HCM, also should be carefully evaluated.[46]

THE ELECTROCARDIOGRAM AS A SCREENING TOOL
Conflicting Recommendations and Controversy

Due to the limited efficacy of the H&P in detecting CVD, as well as the growing appre-ciation of the higher rates of SCA/SCD in competitive athletes, the ECG has garnered interest as a tool to improve the sensitivity of cardiovascular screening. The merits and proposed methods of implementing the ECG as a screening mechanism remain a sub-ject of considerable debate. The European Society of Cardiology (ESC) recommends the routine use of the ECG during cardiovascular preparticipation screening,[55] whereas the AHA does not support ECG screening.[47,56] The AMSSM suggests that ECG screening be considered in higher-risk athletes when accurate ECG interpreta-tion and proper cardiology resources are available.[48] Multiple studies demonstrate that the ECG substantially increases the sensitivity to detect conditions associated with SCA/SCD compared with H&P alone.[51,54,57-59] In a meta-analysis of 15 studies and 47,137 athletes undergoing cardiovascular screening, pooled sensitivities of the screening history, physical examination, and ECG were 20%, 9%, and 94%, respectively.[60]

The Athlete's Heart and Modern Electrocardiogram Interpretation Criteria

It is well established that the hearts of highly trained athletes undergo physiologic ad-aptations due to increased workloads and demand. These changes include ventricular wall hypertrophy and increased vagal tone, known as the athlete's heart.[61] These phys-iologic adaptations can lead to distinct changes on the ECG that can be misinterpreted as pathologic findings by the untrained clinician.[14] The risk of unnecessary restriction of an athlete from participation as a result of misinterpretation, as well as unnecessary secondary testing, is a major criticism of using the ECG as a screening tool.

In order to better distinguish pathologic, disease-specific changes on the ECG from physiologic, athlete's heart changes, athlete-specific ECG criteria have been formu-lated. The first such criteria were published in 2010 by the ESC.[62] Further iterations have followed, including criteria from Stanford University (2011),[63] the Seattle Criteria (2013),[64] the Refined Criteria (2014),[65] and, most recently, the International Criteria

(2017).[14] Each iteration of ECG interpretation criteria has lowered the false-positive rate, or the identification of ECG abnormalities without subsequent diagnosis of disease, without compromising sensitivity to identify underlying cardiac pathology.[66–70] ECG screening by experienced clinicians using athlete-specific standards typically produces false-positive rates of less than 3% to 5%.[51,53] The International Criteria are the current standard for ECG interpretation in athletes,[14] and open access to ECG training modules based on the International Criteria are available at https:// uwsportscardiology.org/e-academy/[71]

Future Screening Directions and Considerations

Screening for any disease by any method carries numerous goals, chiefly

- The detection of a disease in its preclinical course with a high degree of accuracy
- The ability to intervene in order to prevent progression to its clinical state

Although certain H&P findings may suggest the underlying presence of CVD,[46] the exclusive reliance on the H&P for cardiovascular preparticipation screening is considered limited in its ability to detect CVD that places an athlete at elevated risk of SCA/ SCD.[48] The ECG provides a more sensitive screening tool, but skilled sports cardiology infrastructure to conduct accurate interpretation and the appropriate secondary investigations for abnormal ECGs remains limited in the United States. Given the benefits of exercise in young athletes and nonathletes, minimizing unnecessary restriction from participation must also remain a priority, and universal ECG screening of young patients prior to exercise is not recommended by any major medical society. Additional efforts in education and training are needed to provide more effective screening, especially of high-risk athlete subgroups. When deciding on screening methods, consideration of the available sports cardiology resources as well as the risk of an individual athlete based on sport, race, and sex, rather than utilizing an all-or-none approach, is a growing area of interest and may provide a more effective approach.[48,72] Although the ECG is a superior screening tool for the detection of disease, the efficacy of the screening ECG in preventing cardiovascular mortality remains unclear.

HEART DISEASE IN THE ADULT ATHLETE

The cardiovascular care of older athletes (>35 year old) centers on the higher prevalence of atherosclerotic coronary artery disease (CAD) and the potential for exercise-induced acute coronary syndromes stemming from atherosclerotic plaque disruption with thrombosis or fixed stenosis.[73,74] The clinical presentation of these syndromes includes acute myocardial infarction and SCA/SCD, with no preceding symptoms or warning signs in approximately 50% of cases.[75,76] In endurance athletes, oxygen supply and demand mismatch also can precipitate ischemia, infarction, or SCA secondary to a fixed stenosis from a stable plaque (so-called demand ischemia).[77]

Screening in asymptomatic older athletes should focus on CAD risk factor identification and modification and can be carried out well in the primary care setting. Exercise stress testing in asymptomatic, low-risk adults is not recommended by the AHA due to poor predictive values.[78] Furthermore, the American College of Sports Medicine (ACSM) does not recommend the need for specific medical clearance for older athletes who are already participating in moderate to vigorous intensity exercise greater than or equal to 3 days per week, are asymptomatic, and do not carry diagnoses of known cardiovascular, metabolic, or renal disease.[79] Exercise stress testing in adults with 1 or more risk factors for CAD, however, has been shown to have better predictive value and may help inform risk factor modification and interventions.[78] The AHA recommends exercise stress testing prior to the initiation of a vigorous exercise program in men over the age of 45, women over the age of 55, patients with diabetes, and patients with CAD risk factors.[78] The ESC recommends routine exercise stress testing in patients deemed at high risk of CAD,[80] and the ACSM recommends exercise stress testing in high-risk patients prior to the initiation of moderate-intensity or vigorous-intensity exercise programs.[79]

Coronary artery calcium (CAC) scoring by CT shows significant promise in identifying subclinical CAD. Elevated CAC scores are strongly associated with future risk of a cardiovascular event, independent of classic CAD risk factors or symptoms.[81–84] CAC scoring may be appropriate to further risk-stratify patients found to be at intermediate risk of CAD based on standard risk calculators and better inform the selection of candidates for statin therapy.[81,85,86] In 1 study, asymptomatic patients with moderate (100–400) to high ($\geq$400) CAC scores without previously known CAD and who were treated with statin therapy had a lower risk of major cardiovascular events ($P<.05$).[87]

SUMMARY

Heart disease in athletes encompasses a wide variety of conditions and diseases, both congenital and acquired. In the young athlete, the large majority of cases are primary structural or electrical disorders, with SCA/SCD being the most feared, visible, and tragic clinical manifestation. SCA/SCD in young athletes is more common than historically appreciated and can be precipitated in those with any 1 of several conditions. The traditional PPE consists of a screening H&P and is limited in its ability to accurately raise suspicion of underlying CVD. Nevertheless, certain historical clues, especially exertional chest pain or sudden unexplained syncope, should not be discounted and instead prompt further investigations to rule out underlying CVD. ECG screening provides a more sensitive method for the detection of athletes at risk of SCA/SCD but requires a trained sports cardiology infrastructure to conduct accurately. Risk stratification and management strategies for many of the common disorders linked to young athlete SCA/SCD have evolved and in some circumstances allow a return to competitive sport.

In masters athletes, prevention of acute coronary syndromes and SCA precipitated by preexisting CAD is the primary objective. Exercise stress testing in low-risk, asymptomatic patients is not recommended but may be used to guide those with documented risk factors. CAC scoring represents a newer technique to quantify the burden of CAD to risk-stratify patients and may help improve patient-centered outcomes.

DISCLOSURE

The authors have nothing to disclose.

REFERENCES

1. Heron M. Deaths: leading causes for 2016. Natl Vital Stat Rep 2018;67(6):1–77.

2. Harmon KG, Asif IM, Maleszewski JJ, et al. Incidence, cause, and comparative frequency of sudden cardiac death in national collegiate athletic association athletes: a decade in review. Circulation 2015;132(1):10–9.

3. Maron BJ, Doerer JJ, Haas TS, et al. Sudden deaths in young competitive athletes: analysis of 1866 deaths in the United States, 1980-2006. Circulation 2009;119(8):1085–92.
4. Arnett DK, Blumenthal RS, Albert MA, et al. 2019 ACC/AHA guideline on the primary prevention of cardiovascular disease: executive summary: a report of the American College of Cardiology/American Heart Association Task Force on Clinical Practice Guidelines. Circulation 2019;140(11):e463–95.
5. American College of Sports Medicine. Exercise is medicine. 2019. Available at: http://www.exerciseismedicine.org/. Accessed March 28, 2019.
6. Peterson DF, Siebert DM, Kucera KL, et al. Etiology of sudden cardiac arrest and death in US competitive athletes: a 2-year prospective surveillance study. Clin J Sport Med 2018. [Epub ahead of print].
7. Maron BJ, Shirani J, Poliac LC, et al. Sudden death in young competitive athletes. Clinical, demographic, and pathological profiles. JAMA 1996;276(3):199–204.
8. Puranik R, Chow CK, Duflou JA, et al. Sudden death in the young. Heart Rhythm 2005;2(12):1277–82.
9. Holst AG, Winkel BG, Theilade J, et al. Incidence and etiology of sports-related sudden cardiac death in Denmark—implications for preparticipation screening. Heart Rhythm 2010;7(10):1365–71.
10. Papadakis M, Sharma S, Cox S, et al. The magnitude of sudden cardiac death in the young: a death certificate-based review in England and Wales. Europace 2009;11(10):1353–8.
11. Corrado D, Basso C, Pavei A, et al. Trends in sudden cardiovascular death in young competitive athletes after implementation of a preparticipation screening program. JAMA 2006;296(13):1593–601.
12. Maron BJ, Maron MS. Hypertrophic cardiomyopathy. Lancet 2013;381(9862): 242–55.
13. Maron BJ, Roberts WC, Epstein SE. Sudden death in hypertrophic cardiomyopathy: a profile of 78 patients. Circulation 1982;65(7):1388–94.
14. Drezner JA, Sharma S, Baggish A, et al. International criteria for electrocardiographic interpretation in athletes: Consensus statement. Br J Sports Med 2017; 51(9):704–31.
15. Maron BJ, Udelson JE, Bonow RO, et al. Eligibility and disqualification recommendations for competitive athletes with cardiovascular abnormalities: task force 3: hypertrophic cardiomyopathy, arrhythmogenic right ventricular cardiomyopathy and other cardiomyopathies, and myocarditis: a scientific statement from the American Heart Association and American College of Cardiology. Circulation 2015;132(22):273–80.
16. Maron BJ, Rowin EJ, Casey SA, et al. Hypertrophic cardiomyopathy in children, adolescents, and young adults associated with low cardiovascular mortality with contemporary management strategies. Circulation 2016;133(1):62–73.
17. Basso C, Maron BJ, Corrado D, et al. Clinical profile of congenital coronary artery anomalies with origin from the wrong aortic sinus leading to sudden death in young competitive athletes. J Am Coll Cardiol 2000;35(6):1493–501.
18. Edwards CP, Yavari A, Sheppard MN, et al. Anomalous coronary origin: the challenge in preventing exercise-related sudden cardiac death. Br J Sports Med 2010;44(12):895–7.
19. Palmieri V, Gervasi S, Bianco M, et al. Anomalous origin of coronary arteries from the "wrong" sinus in athletes: Diagnosis and management strategies. Int J Cardiol 2018;252:13–20.

20. Pelliccia A, Spataro A, Maron BJ. Prospective echocardiographic screening for coronary artery anomalies in 1,360 elite competitive athletes. Am J Cardiol 1993;72(12):978–9.
21. Van Hare GF, Ackerman MJ, Evangelista JA, et al. Eligibility and disqualification recommendations for competitive athletes with cardiovascular abnormalities: take force 4: congenital heart disease: a scientific statement from the American Heart Association and American College of Cardiology. Circulation 2015; 132(22):e281–91.
22. Cohen MI, Triedman JK, Cannon BC, et al. PACES/HRS expert consensus statement on the management of the asymptomatic young patient with a Wolff-Parkinson-White (WPW, ventricular preexcitation) electrocardiographic pattern: developed in partnership between the Pediatric and Congenital Electrophysiology Society (PACES) and the Heart Rhythm Society (HRS). Endorsed by the governing bodies of PACES, HRS, the American College of Cardiology Foundation (ACCF), the American Heart Association (AHA), the American Academy of Pediatrics (AAP), and the Canadian Heart Rhythm Society (CHRS). Heart Rhythm 2012;9(6):1006–24.
23. Rao AL, Salerno JC, Asif IM, et al. Evaluation and management of Wolff-Parkinson-White in athletes. Sports Health 2014;6(4):326–32.
24. Morita H, Wu J, Zipes DP. The QT syndromes: long and short. Lancet 2008; 372(9640):750–63.
25. Schwartz PJ, Moss AJ, Vincent GM, et al. Diagnostic criteria for the long QT syndrome. Circulation 1993;88(2):782–4.
26. Priori SG, Wilde AA, Horie M, et al. Executive summary: HRS/EHRA/APHRS expert consensus statement on the diagnosis and management of patients with inherited primary arrhythmia syndromes. Heart Rhythm 2013;10(12): e85–108.
27. Pelliccia A, Fagard R, Bjørnstad HH, et al. Recommendations for competitive sports participation in athletes with cardiovascular disease: a consensus document from the Study Group of Sports Cardiology of the Working Group of Cardiac Rehabilitation and Exercise Physiology and the Working Group of Myocardial and Pericardial Diseases of the European Society of Cardiology. Eur Heart J 2005; 26(14):1422–45.
28. Johnson JN, Ackerman MJ. Return to play? Athletes with congenital long QT syndrome. Br J Sports Med 2013;47(1):28–33.
29. Aziz PF, Sweeten T, Vogel RL, et al. Sports participation in genotype positive children with long QT syndrome. JACC Clin Electrophysiol 2015;1(1–2):62–70.
30. Ackerman MJ. Long QT syndrome and sports participation: oil and water or an acceptable and manageable combination? JACC Clin Electrophysiol 2015; 1(1–2):71–3.
31. Ackerman MJ, Zipes DP, Kovacs RJ, et al. Eligibility and disqualification recommendations for competitive athletes with cardiovascular abnormalities: task force 10: the cardiac channelopathies: a scientific statement from the American Heart Association and American College of Cardiology. J Am Coll Cardiol 2015;66(21): 2424–8.
32. Gomez AT, Prutkin JM, Rao AL. Evaluation and management of athletes with long QT syndrome. Sports Health 2016;8(6):527–35.
33. World Anti-Doping Agency. What is prohibited. 2019. Available at: https://www.wada-ama.org/en/content/what-is-prohibited. Accessed April 3, 2019.
34. Zipes DP, Link MS, Ackerman MJ, et al. Eligibility and disqualification recommendations for competitive athletes with cardiovascular abnormalities: task force 9:

arrhythmias and conduction defects: a scientific statement from the American Heart Association and American College of Cardiology. Circulation 2015; 132(22):e315–25.

35. Corrado D, Link MS, Calkins H. Arrhythmogenic right ventricular cardiomyopathy. N Engl J Med 2017;376(1):61–72.

36. McKenna WJ, Thiene G, Nava A, et al. Diagnosis of arrhythmogenic right ventricular dysplasia/cardiomyopathy. Task force of the working group myocardial and pericardial disease of the European Society of Cardiology and of the Scientific Council on Cardiomyopathies of the International Society and Federation of Cardiology. Br Heart J 1994;71(3):215–8.

37. Marcus FI, McKenna WJ, Sherrill D, et al. Diagnosis of arrhythmogenic right ventricular cardiomyopathy/dysplasia: proposed modification of the Task Force Criteria. Eur Heart J 2010;31(7):806–14.

38. Arbustini E, Favalli V, Narula N, et al. Left ventricular noncompaction: a distinct genetic cardiomyopathy? J Am Coll Cardiol 2016;68(9):949–66.

39. Finocchiaro G, Papadakis M, Robertus JL, et al. Etiology of sudden death in sports: insights from a United Kingdom regional registry. J Am Coll Cardiol 2016;67(18):2108–15.

40. Maron BJ, Gohman TE, Aeppli D. Prevalence of sudden cardiac death during competitive sports activities in Minnesota high school athletes. J Am Coll Cardiol 1998;32(7):1881–4.

41. Roberts WO, Stovitz SD. Incidence of sudden cardiac death in Minnesota high school athletes 1993-2012 screened with a standardized pre-participation evaluation. J Am Coll Cardiol 2013;62(14):1298–301.

42. Harmon KG, Drezner JA, Wilson MG, et al. Incidence of sudden cardiac death in athletes: a state-of-the-art review. Br J Sports Med 2014;48(15):1185–92.

43. Steinvil A, Chundadze T, Zeltser D, et al. Mandatory electrocardiographic screening of athletes to reduce their risk for sudden death proven fact or wishful thinking? J Am Coll Cardiol 2011;57(11):1291–6.

44. Drezner JA, Peterson DF, Siebert DM, et al. Survival after exercise-related sudden cardiac arrest in young athletes: can we do better? Sports Health 2019; 11(1):91–8.

45. Harmon KG, Asif IM, Klossner D, et al. Incidence of sudden cardiac death in National Collegiate Athletic Association athletes. Circulation 2011;123(15): 1594–600.

46. American Academy of Family Physicians, American Academy of Pediatrics, American College of Sports Medicine, et al. Preparticipation physical evaluation. 4th edition. Itasca, IL: American Academy of Pediatrics; 2010.

47. Maron BJ, Friedman RA, Kligfield P, et al. Assessment of the 12-lead electrocardiogram as a screening test for detection of cardiovascular disease in healthy general populations of young people (12-25 years of age): a scientific statement from the American Heart Association and the American College of Cardiology. J Am Coll Cardiol 2014;64(14):1479–514.

48. Drezner JA, O'Connor FG, Harmon KG, et al. AMSSM position statement on cardiovascular preparticipation screening in athletes: current evidence, knowledge gaps, recommendations and future directions. Br J Sports Med 2017;51(3): 153–67.

49. Carrado D, Basso C, Rizzoli G, et al. Does sports activity enhance the risk of sudden death in adolescents and young adults? J Am Coll Cardiol 2003;42(11): 1959–63.

50. Hainline B, Drezner JA, Baggish A, et al. Interassociation consensus statement on cardiovascular care of college student-athletes. Br J Sports Med 2017; 51(2):74–85.
51. Fudge J, Harmon KG, Owens DS, et al. Cardiovascular screening in adolescents and young adults: a prospective study comparing the Pre-participation Physical Evaluation Monograph 4th Edition and ECG. Br J Sports Med 2014;48(15): 1172–8.
52. Zeltser I, Cannon B, Silvana L, et al. Lessons learned from preparticipation cardiovascular screening in a state funded program. Am J Cardiol 2012;110(6): 902–8.
53. Drezner JA, Prutkin JM, Harmon KG, et al. Cardiovascular screening in college athletes. J Am Coll Cardiol 2015;65(21):2353–5.
54. Drezner JA, Owens DS, Prutkin JM, et al. Electrocardiographic screening in national collegiate athletic association athletes. Am J Cardiol 2016;118(5):754–9.
55. Corrado D, Pelliccia A, Bjørnstad HH, et al. Cardiovascular pre-participation screening of young competitive athletes for prevention of sudden death: proposal for a common European protocol. Consensus statement of the study group of sport cardiology of the working group of cardiac rehabilitation and exercise physiology and the working group of myocardial and pericardial diseases of the European Society of Cardiology. Eur Heart J 2005;26(5):516–24.
56. Maron BJ, Thompson PD, Ackerman MJ, et al. Recommendations and considerations related to preparticipation screening for cardiovascular abnormalities in competitive athletes: 2007 update: a scientific statement from the American Heart Association Council on Nutrition, Physical Activity, and Metabolism: endorsed by the American College of Cardiology Foundation. Circulation 2007;115(12): 1643–55.
57. Price DE, McWilliams A, Asif IM, et al. Electrocardiography-inclusive screening strategies for detection of cardiovascular abnormalities in high school athletes. Heart Rhythm 2014;11(3):442–9.
58. Fuller CM, McNulty CM, Spring DA, et al. Prospective screening of 5,615 high school athletes for risk of sudden cardiac death. Med Sci Sports Exerc 1997; 29(9):1131–8.
59. Wilson MG, Basavarajaiah S, Whyte GP, et al. Efficacy of personal symptom and family history questionnaires when screening for inherited cardiac pathologies: the role of electrocardiography. Br J Sports Med 2008;42(3):207–11.
60. Harmon KG, Zigman M, Drezner JA, et al. The effectiveness of screening history, physical exam, and ECG to detect potentially lethal cardiac disorders in athletes: a systematic review/meta-analysis. J Electrocardiol 2015;48(3):329–38.
61. Maron BJ, Pelliccia A, Spirito P. Cardiac disease in young trained athletes. Insights into methods for distinguishing athlete's heart from structural heart disease, with particular emphasis on hypertrophic cardiomyopathy. Circulation 1995;91(5):1596–601.
62. Corrado D, Pelliccia A, Heidbuchel H, et al. Recommendations for interpretation of 12-lead electrocardiogram in the athlete. Eur Heart J 2010;31(2):243–59.
63. Uberoi A, Stein R, Perez MV, et al. Interpretation of the electrocardiogram of young athletes. Circulation 2011;124(6):746–57.
64. Drezner JA, Ackerman MJ, Anderson J, et al. Electrocardiographic interpretation in athletes: the 'Seattle Criteria'. Br J Sports Med 2013;47(3):122–4.
65. Sheikh N, Papadakis M, Ghani S, et al. Comparison of electrocardiographic criteria for the detection of cardiac abnormalities in elite black and white athletes. Circulation 2014;129(16):1637–49.

66. Brosnan M, La Gerche A, Kalman J, et al. The Seattle Criteria increase the specificity of preparticipation ECG screening among elite athletes. Br J Sports Med 2014;48(15):1144–50.
67. Riding NR, Sheikh N, Adamuz C, et al. Comparison of three current sets of electrocardiographic interpretation criteria for use in screening athletes. Heart 2015; 101(5):384–90.
68. Fuller C, Scott C, Hug-English C, et al. Five-year experience with screening electrocardiograms in national collegiate athletic association division I athletes. Clin J Sport Med 2016;26(5):369–75.
69. Zorzi A, Calore C, Vio R, et al. Accuracy of the ECG for differential diagnosis between hypertrophic cardiomyopathy and athlete's heart: comparison between the European Society of Cardiology (2010) and International (2017) criteria. Br J Sports Med 2018;52(10):667–73.
70. McClean G, Riding NR, Pieles G, et al. Diagnostic accuracy and Bayesian analysis of new international ECG recommendations in paediatric athletes. Heart 2019;105(2):152–9.
71. UW Medicine Center For Sports Cardiology, Australasian College of Sport and Exercise Physicians. ECG interpretation in athletes. 2019. Available at: https://uwsportscardiology.org/e-academy/. Accessed April 12, 2019.
72. Drezner JA, Harmon KG, Asif IM, et al. Why cardiovascular screening in young athletes can save lives: a critical review. Br J Sports Med 2016;50(22):1376–8.
73. Giri S, Thompson PD, Kiernan FJ, et al. Clinical and angiographic characteristics of exertion-related acute myocardial infarction. JAMA 1999;282(18):1731–6.
74. Thompson PD. Exercise prescription and proscription for patients with coronary artery disease. Circulation 2005;112(15):2354–63.
75. Marijon E, Uy-Evanado A, Dumas F, et al. Warning symptoms are associated with survival from sudden cardiac arrest. Ann Intern Med 2016;164(1):23–9.
76. Nehme Z, Bernard S, Andrew E, et al. Warning symptoms preceding out-of-hospital cardiac arrest: Do patient delays matter? Resuscitation 2018;123:65–70.
77. Kim JH, Malhotra R, Chiampas G, et al. Cardiac arrest during long-distance running races. N Engl J Med 2012;366(2):130–40.
78. Fletcher GF, Ades PA, Kligfield P, et al. Exercise standards for testing and training: a scientific statement from the American Heart Association. Circulation 2013;128(8):873–934.
79. Riebe D, Franklin BA, Thompson PD, et al. Updating ACSM's recommendations for exercise preparticipation health screening. Med Sci Sports Exerc 2015; 47(11):2473–9.
80. Mont L, Pelliccia A, Sharma S, et al. Pre-participation cardiovascular evaluation for athletic participants to prevent sudden death: Position paper from the EHRA and the EACPR, branches of the ESC. Endorsed by APHRS, HRS, and SOLAECE. Eur J Prev Cardiol 2017;24(1):41–69.
81. Hecht HS, Cronin P, Blaha MJ, et al. 2016 SCCT/STR guidelines for coronary artery calcium scoring of noncontrast noncardiac chest CT scans: a report of the Society of Cardiovascular Computed Tomography and Society of Thoracic Radiology. J Thorac Imaging 2017;32(5):W54–66.
82. Carr JJ, Jacobs DR Jr, Terry JG, et al. Association of coronary artery calcium in adults aged 32 to 46 years with incident coronary heart disease and death. JAMA Cardiol 2017;2(4):391–9.
83. Budoff MJ, Young R, Burke G, et al. Ten-year association of coronary artery calcium with atherosclerotic cardiovascular disease (ASCVD) events: the multiethnic study of atherosclerosis (MESA). Eur Heart J 2018;39(25):2401–8.

84. Mitchell JD, Paisley R, Moon P, et al. Coronary artery calcium and long-term risk of death, myocardial infarction, and stroke: the walter reed cohort study. JACC Cardiovasc Imaging 2018;11(12):1799–806.
85. Lloyd-Jones DM, Braun LT, Ndumele CE, et al. Use of risk assessment tools to guide decision-making in the primary prevention of atherosclerotic cardiovascular disease: a special report from the American Heart Association and American College of Cardiology. J Am Coll Cardiol 2019;73(24):3153–67.
86. Wolk MJ, Bailey SR, Doherty JU, et al. ACCF/AHA/ASE/ASNC/HFSA/HRS/SCAI/ SCCT/SCMR/STS 2013 multimodality appropriate use criteria for the detection and risk assessment of stable ischemic heart disease: a report of the American College of Cardiology Foundation Appropriate Use Criteria Task Force, American Heart Association, American Society of Echocardiography, American Society of Nuclear Cardiology, Heart Failure Society of America, Heart Rhythm Society, Society for Cardiovascular Angiography and Interventions, Society of Cardiovascular Computed Tomography, Society for Cardiovascular Magnetic Resonance, and Society of Thoracic Surgeons. J Am Coll Cardiol 2014;63(4):380–406.
87. Mitchell JD, Fergestrom N, Gage BF, et al. Impact of statins on cardiovascular outcomes following coronary artery calcium scoring. J Am Coll Cardiol 2018; 72(25):3233–42.

Sports Supplements
Pearls and Pitfalls

Katherine M. Edenfield, MD

KEYWORDS

- Sports supplement • Sport foods • Medical supplements • Ergogenic supplements
- Supplement resources • DHSEA act

KEY POINTS

- Supplements are not regulated by the US Food and Drug Administration.
- They may get to the market and be contaminated with substances banned in sport or dangerous to health, and the contents may not contain what is listed on the label.
- Sports supplements can be generally divided into 3 categories: sports foods (foods/drinks containing macronutrients), medical supplements (vitamins/minerals used to treat deficiencies), and ergogenic supplements (used to benefit performance).
- There are third-party companies that provide certification to supplements of label verification, quality, integrity, and presence of contaminants and banned substances for sport.
- When choosing to use a supplement, the safest practice is to choose a certified brand.

INTRODUCTION

There are many different definitions of the term "dietary supplement." The Dietary Supplement Health and Education Act of 1994 defines a dietary supplement as a product taken by mouth that contains a "dietary ingredient" intended to supplement the diet.[1] The "dietary ingredients" in these products may include vitamins, minerals, herbs or other botanicals, amino acids, and substances such as enzymes, organ tissues, glandulars, and metabolites. Dietary supplements can also be extracts or concentrates, and may be found in many forms such as tablets, capsules, soft gels, gel caps, liquids, or powders.[1] Dietary supplements must contain a "dietary ingredient" and not contain drugs. Drugs are distinct in that they are intended to treat, diagnose, prevent, or cure disease. Supplements are not and may not make these claims.[2] Under the Dietary Supplement Health and Education Act, the US Food and Drug Administration (FDA) has no authority to approve dietary supplements for safety or effectiveness before they reach consumers.[3] Once marketed, the FDA can take action to remove products from the market, but first must prove that the product is either

Department of Community Health and Family Medicine, University of Florida, Student Health Care Center, 280 Fletcher Drive, PO Box 117500, Gainesville, FL 32611, USA
E-mail address: kedenfield@ufl.edu

Prim Care Clin Office Pract 47 (2020) 37–48
https://doi.org/10.1016/j.pop.2019.10.002
0095-4543/20/© 2019 Elsevier Inc. All rights reserved.

primarycare.theclinics.com

unsafe or misbranded (ie, has false or misleading labeling).[2] The process to get a supplement off the market is usually long and complicated. It takes time for the FDA to identify unsafe or adulterated (containing unapproved ingredients) supplements postmarket, because they have to rely on review of adverse event reports, consumer complaints, inspection of dietary supplement firms, and screening of imported products.[4] True adverse events are likely underreported owing to both consumers and physicians not attributing the symptoms to the dietary supplement or knowing how to report.[4] Once an unsafe or adulterated supplement is identified, the FDA issues a warning, which can include a voluntary recall from the responsible dietary supplement firm, public notification, news release, consumer update, or warning letter to the firm.[4] One study looking at 9 years of adulterated dietary supplements found that 46.4% had a voluntary recall by the dietary supplement firm and 44.1% were associated with a public notification only.[4] For example, 1,3-dimethylamylamine (DMAA) is an amphetamine derivative ingredient that can be found in dietary supplements. After several active duty military soldiers died after taking supplements with DMAA in 2012,[5] the FDA issued warning letters to companies with DMAA in their products notifying them the products violated the law.[6] In 2013, the FDA detained 2 DMAA-containing products after they refused to comply with voluntarily recalling their products; the parent company ultimately destroyed the products.[6] Also in 2013, the FDA seized DMAA-containing products from another company; in 2017, a federal district court ruled the products were adulterated and should be destroyed. This case is currently on appeal.[6] The FDA has issued warning letters to companies regarding DMAA in their products as recently as October 2017.[6]

Athletes of all types and levels use supplements. Reasons include fueling, recovery, to aid performance, and to treat deficiencies. One study of elite Australian swimmers reported 97% had used supplements or sports food in the previous year.[7] Another study of high-performance Canadian athletes reported 87% had used 3 or more supplements in the previous 6 months.[8]

For the purposes of this review, we categorize nutritional supplements into 3 categories to include sports foods (gels, bars, drinks, protein powders), medical supplements (vitamins and minerals used to treat clinical deficiency or problem), and ergogenic supplements (used to benefit performance).

SPORT FOODS
Sports Drink

Typical composition
Liquid containing 5% to 8% carbohydrate, 10 to 35 mmol/L sodium, and 3 to 5 mmol/L potassium.[9]

Common sports-related use
During exercise lasting longer than 60 minutes to replace depleted glycogen stores and alleviate hypoglycemia, improving endurance performance, and to replete glycogen stores following a workout or competition. For maximal effectiveness, a carbohydrate intake of 1 g/min at 15- to 30-minute intervals would start 30 minutes before blood glucose levels start to decline. Electrolyte addition maintains osmotic drive for drinking during recovery and enhances palatability leading to better hydration.[10]

Sports Bar

Typical composition
Sports bars typically contain 40 to 50 g carbohydrate, 5 to 10 g protein, low in fat and fiber, and other vitamins/minerals up to 100% of the recommended daily allowance.[9]

Common sports-related use
Easy and on-the-go nutrition, postexercise recovery, and during exercise carbohydrate source.

Sports Gel

Typical composition
Sports gel typically contain 20 to 25 g carbohydrate, 1 to 4%DV of sodium and potassium, and no protein or fat. Some may contain caffeine or related substances.

Common sports-related use
During exercise as an easily absorbed carbohydrate source. Need to take with water.

Protein Supplement

Typical composition
Protein supplements typically contain 20 to 40 g protein dose in powder or liquid form, usually containing whey, casein, and milk and egg proteins. Acute protein doses should contain 700 to 3000 mg of leucine in addition to a balanced array of the essential amino acids.[11]

Common sports-related use
To stimulate muscle protein synthesis, synergistic with exercise stimulus when protein consumption occurs before or after resistance exercise.[12] To build and maintain muscle mass.

MEDICAL SUPPLEMENTS
Vitamin D

Overview
Vitamin D is a fat-soluble vitamin obtained from UVB light, foods, and supplementation which is initially biologically inert until it undergoes hydroxylation first in the liver to calcidiol (25-hydroxyvitamin D) followed by a second hydroxylation in the kidney to the physiologically active form of Vitamin D known as calcitriol (1,25 dihydroxyvitamin D).[13] It promotes calcium absorption in the gut, enables normal mineralization of bone, aids in bone growth and remodeling, and has roles in neuromuscular and immune function.[13] Serum 25-hydroxyvitamin D [25(OH)D] levels are the best indicator of vitamin D status as it reflects that produced cutaneously and obtained orally and has a half-life of 15 days. Calcitriol has a 15-hour half-life and is closely regulated by other hormones and minerals in the body.[13]

Typical supplementation protocol
No consensus over the definition of vitamin D deficiency. In athletes a value of less than 30 ng/mL (75 nmol/L) is often used.[14] Supplementation for deficiency is typically 50,000 IU of vitamin D_3 per week for 8 to 12 weeks. Peak neuromuscular performance is associated with 25(OH)D, calcidiol, levels of 50 ng/mL with no apparent added benefits above that level.[14] Supplementation of between 800 IU and 2000 IU/day is recommended to maintain optimal status for general population.[9]

Effectiveness
Supplementation of vitamin D to a sufficient level (>30 ng/mL) in combination with calcium is effective in optimizing bone health by increasing bone mineral density and reducing fractures in elderly institutionalized populations.[13] There is currently not adequate evidence of vitamin D being effective in other conditions or in exercise performance.[11,13] There is a growing body of research that optimal vitamin D levels

decrease incidence and severity of upper respiratory tract infections by improving immune function[15]

Possible adverse effects
Acute toxicity [serum 25(OH)D levels of 200–240 ng/mL] can lead to anorexia, weight loss, polyuria, arrhythmias, vascular and tissue calcifications, and kidney stones.[13] Possible adverse health effects over time from lower serum levels (50–60 ng/mL) include increase in all-cause mortality, a greater risk of certain types of cancer, an increased risk of cardiovascular events, and more falls and fractures among the elderly. Based on these data, the tolerable upper intake levels of vitamin D for adults is 4000 IU/d.[13]

Iron

Iron is an essential mineral component of hemoglobin in the red blood cell that is necessary for oxygen delivery throughout the body in addition to other roles in metabolism, respiration, and immune function.[16] Suboptimal iron levels may occur from poor intake, bioavailability, increased need from growth, high altitude training, menstrual blood loss, foot-strike hemolysis, or increased loss in sweat, urine, and feces.[9] Ferritin is generally reflective of total body iron stores, and therefore generally used for screening for iron deficiency. However, it is also an acute phase reactant and will not be an accurate marker in individuals with any systemic inflammation.

Typical supplementation protocol
Very inconsistent in the literature owing to lack of consistency and agreement on a ferritin level that is considered deficient. A recent review found that a ferritin cutoff of 20 μg/L may be reasonable as the point at which to consider iron supplementation for performance improvement for iron-deficient nonanemic athletes.[16] Ferrous sulfate (20% elemental iron) is the most frequently used and widely available iron supplement. One 100 to 325 mg dose per day of ferrous sulfate would be reasonable in an iron-deficient nonanemic athlete. In an iron-deficient anemic athlete, a higher dose would be indicated.

Effectiveness
Iron seems to be of no benefit as a supplement to achieve serum ferritin levels of greater than 20 μg/L,[16] but there may be a performance benefit to supplement iron in athletes with serum ferritins of less than 20 μg/L. A randomized controlled trial in female rowers found that supplementation improved ferritin levels during training, decreased energy expenditure, increased energy efficiency, and slowed the lactate response during a 4-km time trial.[17] Impact on actual race performance is unknown and difficult to assess.

Possible adverse effects
Nausea, vomiting, constipation, dark stools, dyspepsia.

Probiotics

Probiotics are live micro-organisms (bacteria and yeast). Certain probiotics can confer health benefits to the consumer, when administered in a viable form and in adequate amounts. The most common probiotics are *Lactobacillus* and *Bifidobacterium* species.

Typical supplementation protocol
A typical dose is 10^{10} live bacteria daily.

Effectiveness

A 2015 Cochrane review showed probiotics were better than placebo in decreasing the number of upper respiratory tract infections by 47% and the duration of an acute upper respiratory tract infection by 1.89 days.[18] Another study looked specifically at probiotic supplementation in athletes over 4 months of winter training and found a 36% decrease in upper respiratory tract infection symptoms, and a significantly higher salivary IgA concentration, with athletes taking a *Lactobacillus* probiotic than those taking placebo.[19] There is also evidence for probiotic supplementation preventing diarrhea, eczema in children, and improving cardiometabolic parameters in patients with type 2 diabetes.[20]

Possible adverse effects

Minor gastrointestinal side effects. A 2011 report released by the Agency for Healthcare Research and Quality that reviewed 622 studies of organisms from *Lactobacillus*, *Bifidobacterium*, *Saccaromyces*, *Streptococcus*, *Enterococcus*, and *Bacillus* and found no evidence of increased risk, but that the current literature is not sufficient to report confidently on the safety of probiotics, because the majority of studies did not assess or report safety.[21] Patients at higher risk of adverse events include immunocompromised patients, premature infants, those with short bowel syndrome or central venous catheters, and those with cardiac valve disease.[22]

Omega-3 Fatty Acids

Omega-3 fatty acids (FAs) are found in fish oil in the form of eicosapentaenoic acid and docosahexaenoic acid (DHA). Salmon, tuna, mackerel, herring, sardines, and anchovies contain some of the highest levels of fish oil. Alpha-linolenic acid is a vegetable source of omega-3 FA, but does not have all of the same health benefits eicosapentaenoic acid and DHA do.

Typical supplementation protocol

A 1 to 2 g/d dose at a ratio of eicosapentaenoic acid to DHA of 2:1 for counteracting exercise-induced inflammation and for overall health. The FDA has designated 3 g/d or less as safe.[23] Human clinical trials are pending regarding use and dosing for concussion, but translating the dose used in rat studies equals an estimated intake of about 387 mg/d of DHA.[23]

Effectiveness

In athletics, there is considerable interest in the use of omega-3 FAs in mild traumatic brain injury. Omega-3 FAs have important structural and functional roles in the central nervous system. DHA is the predominant omega-3 FA in the brain and most important to brain development and cognitive function. There is promising evidence that DHA may help as a recovery aid, partially by mitigating oxidative stress, or as a prophylactic measure in mild traumatic brain injury.[24] Omega-3 FAs have also been used for their anti-inflammatory effects. One study showed that participants taking 3 g of fish oil per day for 6 weeks had decreased markers of oxidative stress after a single bout of eccentric exercise, but no difference in muscle soreness.[25] The cumulative current data are currently inconclusive on whether omega 3 FAs effectively attenuate the inflammatory and immunomodulatory response to exercise or is ergogenic.[23]

Possible adverse effects

There is some concern that a high dose (>3 g/d) can potentially increase bleeding risk and suppress immune response.[26] Fish oil supplements can cause a fishy aftertaste or "fishy burp." Fish oil can also cause halitosis, heartburn, dyspepsia, nausea, loose stools, and rash.

ERGOGENIC SUPPLEMENTS

See **Table 1** for an overview of ergogenic supplements.

Caffeine

Caffeine is a stimulant frequently used by athletes for ergogenic effects. Proposed ergogenic effects are through 3 mechanisms of action: an increased mobilization of intracellular calcium, an increase in free FA oxidation, and serving as an adenosine receptor antagonist in the central nervous system, which may modulate central fatigue, decrease ratings of perceived exertion and pain, and improving levels of vigor.[27]

Typical supplementation protocol
Three to 6 mg/kg/body weight (no benefit seen after 6 mg/kg) less than 60 minutes before competition and if practical, during competition. Athletes should abstain from caffeine at least 7 days before competition to allow adenosine receptor downregulation to occur before ergogenic use.[27]

Effectiveness
There is good evidence for improved endurance capacity, increasing time to fatigue and time trial activities from 5 to 150 minutes' duration across a wide range of exercises.[27,28] Cycling time trial performance was improved 3% to 7% (more with higher doses of caffeine) in one study.[29] Caffeine has also been shown effective in short duration high-intensity exercise, improving performance time, mean speed and power, and peak power in a cycling time trial of 1 to 2 minutes' duration,[30] as well as repeated, intermittent team sport sprinting activity.[31]

Possible adverse effects
Anxiety, insomnia, restlessness, nausea, arrhythmias, hypertension, tremor, headache, diarrhea.

Table 1
Ergogenic supplements: typical supplementation protocols and efficacy

Ergogenic Supplement	Typical Protocol	Effectiveness
Caffeine	3–6 mg/kg/body weight <60 min before competition	Yes, for increasing endurance capacity, increasing time to fatigue, and time trial activities 5–150 min
Creatine monohydrate	Load 5 g (0.3 g/kg/body weight) 4×s daily × 5–7 d followed by maintenance phase 3–5 g/d as a single dose	Yes, for single and repetitive short-term (<30s) high intensity tasks
Beta Alanine	3.2–6.4 g/d in divided doses of 0.8–1.6 g every 3–4 h × 4–12 wk	Probably, in improving exercise capacity for exercises between 0.5–10 min
Nitrate	8.4 mmol (520 mg) from nitrate-rich beetroot juice 2–3 h before performance	Probably, if dosed appropriately for high-intensity repeat sprint performance between 12–40 min duration

Creatine

Creatine is a nitrogen compound synthesized in the pancreas and liver from the amino acids glycine, arginine, and methionine. Approximately 95% is stored in skeletal muscle, of that two-thirds is phosphocreatine and the remaining amount is stored as free creatine. Used to rephosphorylate adenosine diphosphate to adenosine triphosphate during and after intense exercise. The ability to sustain high-intensity exercise diminishes as phosphocreatine stores are depleted owing to decreased energy availability.[32] Supplementation increases phosphocreatine stores, a key substrate for high-intensity force generation, enhancing both single and repeated bouts of short-term, high-intensity efforts.[33] The chronic training adaptations related to enhanced high-intensity training also leads to increased lean mass and muscular strength and power.[33]

Typical supplementation protocol

Creatine is given as a loading phase of approximately 5 g (0.3 g/kg body weight) of creatine monohydrate 4 times daily for 5 to 7 days followed by a maintenance phase of single dose of 3 to 5 g/d. Consumption with a concurrent carbohydrate with or without a protein source may promote greater muscle creatine uptake.[34]

Effectiveness

Creatine is effective for performance enhancements for single and repetitive short-term (<30 seconds) high-intensity exercise tasks (sprints, strength, and power activities) in both upper and lower body activities.[33,35,36]

Possible adverse effects

Creatine is very safe. No negative health effects in a cohort of athletes taking creatine for up to 4 years at recommended loading and maintenance doses.[37] A potential 1- to 3-kg increase in body mass does occur with creatine loading owing to an increase in total body water,[38] which may be undesirable in certain sports. There is no evidence that creatine contributes to muscle cramps or dehydration, and it may actually enhance performance in the heat through improved thermoregulation, among other mechanisms.[38]

Beta-Alanine

Beta-alanine is a nonessential amino acid produced endogenously in the liver and is the rate-limiting factor to the intramuscular synthesis of carnosine, which is an intracellular buffer. It is supplemented in an effort to improve muscular buffering capacity to decrease intramuscular acidosis, a contributing factor to fatigue.[39]

Typical supplementation protocol

Beta-alanine is given as 3.2 to 6.4 g/d in divided doses of 0.8 to 1.6 g every 3 to 4 hours to minimize side effects for 4 to 12 weeks.[40]

Effectiveness

Beta-alanine seems to be effective in improving exercise capacity for exercises lasting between 0.5 and 10.0 minutes.[41] There is an unclear effect on actual competition performance in elite swimmers.[41] Co-supplementation with sodium bicarbonate can provide additive gains.[39,40]

Possible adverse effects

Paresthesia is the only known side effect, caused by acute plasma elevation of beta-alanine after a single dose.[39] This effect can be decreased through dividing the total daily dose throughout the day.[39]

Nitrate

Dietary nitrate can help to decrease the oxygen cost of submaximal exercise, improve exercise tolerance, and enhance repeated sprint performance via its reduction to nitrite and nitric oxide and their physiologic and functional responses in type II muscle fibers.[42–44]

Typical supplementation protocol

Usually taken as either beetroot juice or sodium nitrate. Acutely, 8.4 mmol (520 mg) of nitrate-rich beetroot juice (approximately 4.1 mmol/70 mL) is taken 2 to 3 hours before performance to improve O_2 uptake during moderate intensity exercise and increase time-to-task failure.[45] More chronic daily supplementation with 6 mmol for up to 4 weeks can reduce the oxygen cost of submaximal exercise,[44] whereas 12.8 mmol of daily nitrate in beetroot juice for 7 days enhanced repeated sprint performance.[43]

Effectiveness

Nitrate seems to be dose and timing dependent. Doses listed in supplementation protocol described were found to be most effective than lower doses studied. It is also possible that trained athletes require a larger dose of nitrate, or a chronic supplementation strategy, than their relatively untrained counterparts to see performance benefits.[46] Nitrate seems to be beneficial for high-intensity repeat sprint performance between 12 to 40 minutes' duration with shorter recovery intervals (20–24seconds) than for longer duration intervals or a longer recovery is expected.[43,47]

Possible adverse effects

Nitrate is not carcinogenic, but if ingested under conditions that result in endogenous nitrosation (reaction of nitrite sources with amino compounds), it may lead to an increased cancer risk.[48]

DIETARY SUPPLEMENT RESOURCES
Independent Third-Party Tested and Certified

Some companies choose to certify their supplements. In general, a certified supplement indicates that:

- Contents of the supplement match what is on the label
- There are no unsafe levels of contaminants (ie, heavy metals)
- Manufactured at a facility that uses FDA current Good Manufacturing Practices

In addition, some also include a "sport" version of their certification which also tests and cross-references to make sure that the products do not contain any substances banned by major athletic organizations. Examples of these certifications are listed here:

National Science Foundation certified for sport[49]
Banned Substance Control Group[50]
United States Pharmacopeia[51]
Informed-Choice.org[52]

Other Resources

In addition, other helpful resources when it comes to supplements are:

- The Natural Medicine Sports Medicine Database[53] (requires subscription), which has a comprehensive review of individual supplements/herbals with regard to efficacy, dosing, and adverse effects.

- The Consumer Lab[54] (requires subscription), which independently tests and compares certain supplements and reports results to consumers.
- The United States Anti-Doping Agency has a resource called Supplement 411[55] on their website full of resources regarding supplements for athletes and practitioners.
- The FDA[56] has a resource on their website on dietary supplements and provides consumer alerts that provide an option to subscribe to.

ADVICE TO PATIENTS

- It is best practice to always choose food over dietary supplements. Food contains numerous nutrients together that may not work as well individually when isolated. Supplements cannot compensate for poor dietary habits and do not contain all the nutrients found in food.
- Supplements are not regulated by the FDA and may be contaminated or not contain the ingredients listed on the label.
- If the benefits of a supplement seem to outweigh the risks; do your research and choose a reputable source.

DISCLOSURE

The author has nothing to disclose.

REFERENCES

1. Administration USFaD. Questions and answers on dietary supplements. 2017. Available at: https://www.fda.gov/Food/DietarySupplements/UsingDietarySupplements/ucm480069.htm#what_is. Accessed June 12, 2018.

2. Administration USFaD. Dietary supplement products and ingredients. 2017. Available at: https://www.fda.gov/Food/DietarySupplements/ProductsIngredients/default.htm. Accessed June 12, 2018.

3. Adminstration USFaD. Information for consumers on using dietary supplements. 2018. Available at: https://www.fda.gov/Food/DietarySupplements/UsingDietarySupplements/default.htm. Accessed June 12, 2018.

4. Tucker J, Fischer T, Upjohn L, et al. Unapproved pharmaceutical ingredients included in dietary supplements associated with US Food and Drug Administration warnings. JAMA Netw Open 2018;1(6):e183337.

5. Eliason MJ, Eichner A, Cancio A, et al. Case reports: death of active duty soldiers following ingestion of dietary supplements containing 1,3-dimethylamylamine (DMAA). Mil Med 2012;177(12):1455–9.

6. FDA) USFaDA. DMAA in products marketed as dietary supplements 2018. Available at: https://www.fda.gov/food/dietary-supplement-products-ingredients/dmaa-products-marketed-dietary-supplements. Accessed May 7, 2019.

7. Shaw G, Slater G, Burke LM. Supplement use of elite Australian swimmers. Int J Sport Nutr Exerc Metab 2016;26(3):249–58.

8. Lun V, Erdman KA, Fung TS, et al. Dietary supplementation practices in Canadian high-performance athletes. Int J Sport Nutr Exerc Metab 2012;22(1):31–7.

9. Maughan RJ, Burke LM, Dvorak J, et al. IOC consensus statement: dietary supplements and the high-performance athlete. Int J Sport Nutr Exerc Metab 2018;28(2):104–25.

10. Marriott BM, Institute of Medicine (U.S.). Committee on military nutrition research. Fluid replacement and heat stress. Washington, DC: National Academy Press; 1994. Available at: http://www.ncbi.nlm.nih.gov/books/NBK231130/.

11. Kerksick CM, Wilborn CD, Roberts MD, et al. ISSN exercise & sports nutrition review update: research & recommendations. J Int Soc Sports Nutr 2018;15(1):38.

12. Jäger R, Kerksick CM, Campbell BI, et al. International Society of Sports Nutrition Position Stand: protein and exercise. J Int Soc Sports Nutr 2017;14:20.

13. Vitamin D: fact sheet for health professionals. 2018. Available at: https://ods.od.nih.gov/factsheets/VitaminD-HealthProfessional/.

14. Shuler FD, Wingate MK, Moore GH, et al. Sports health benefits of vitamin D. Sports Health 2012;4(6):496–501.

15. Owens DJ, Allison R, Close GL. Vitamin D and the athlete: current perspectives and new challenges. Sports Med 2018;48(Suppl 1):3–16.

16. Rubeor A, Goojha C, Manning J, et al. Does iron supplementation improve performance in iron-deficient nonanemic athletes? Sports Health 2018;10(5):400–5.

17. DellaValle DM, Haas JD. Iron supplementation improves energetic efficiency in iron-depleted female rowers. Med Sci Sports Exerc 2014;46(6):1204–15.

18. Hao Q, Dong BR, Wu T. Probiotics for preventing acute upper respiratory tract infections. Cochrane Database Syst Rev 2015;(2):CD006895.

19. Gleeson M, Bishop NC, Oliveira M, et al. Daily probiotic's (Lactobacillus casei Shirota) reduction of infection incidence in athletes. Int J Sport Nutr Exerc Metab 2011;21(1):55–64.

20. Valdes AM, Walter J, Segal E, et al. Role of the gut microbiota in nutrition and health. BMJ 2018;361:k2179.

21. Hempel S, Newberry S, Ruelaz A, et al. Safety of probiotics used to reduce risk and prevent or treat disease. Evid Rep Technol Assess (Full Rep) 2011;(200):1–645.

22. Doron S, Snydman DR. Risk and safety of probiotics. Clin Infect Dis 2015;60(Suppl 2):S129–34.

23. Shei RJ, Lindley MR, Mickleborough TD. Omega-3 polyunsaturated fatty acids in the optimization of physical performance. Mil Med 2014;179(11 Suppl):144–56.

24. Barrett EC, McBurney MI, Ciappio ED. ω-3 fatty acid supplementation as a potential therapeutic aid for the recovery from mild traumatic brain injury/concussion. Adv Nutr 2014;5(3):268–77.

25. Gray P, Chappell A, Jenkinson AM, et al. Fish oil supplementation reduces markers of oxidative stress but not muscle soreness after eccentric exercise. Int J Sport Nutr Exerc Metab 2014;24(2):206–14.

26. Mickleborough TD. Omega-3 polyunsaturated fatty acids in physical performance optimization. Int J Sport Nutr Exerc Metab 2013;23(1):83–96.

27. Ganio MS, Klau JF, Casa DJ, et al. Effect of caffeine on sport-specific endurance performance: a systematic review. J Strength Cond Res 2009;23(1):315–24.

28. Burke LM. Caffeine and sports performance. Appl Physiol Nutr Metab 2008;33(6):1319–34.

29. Talanian JL, Spriet LL. Low and moderate doses of caffeine late in exercise improve performance in trained cyclists. Appl Physiol Nutr Metab 2016;41(8):850–5.

30. Wiles JD, Coleman D, Tegerdine M, et al. The effects of caffeine ingestion on performance time, speed and power during a laboratory-based 1 km cycling time-trial. J Sports Sci 2006;24(11):1165–71.

31. Wellington BM, Leveritt MD, Kelly VG. The effect of caffeine on repeat-high-intensity-effort performance in rugby league players. Int J Sports Physiol Perform 2017;12(2):206–10.
32. Buford TW, Kreider RB, Stout JR, et al. International Society of Sports Nutrition position stand: creatine supplementation and exercise. J Int Soc Sports Nutr 2007; 4:6.
33. Peeling P, Binnie MJ, Goods PSR, et al. Evidence-based supplements for the enhancement of athletic performance. Int J Sport Nutr Exerc Metab 2018;28(2): 178–87.
34. Kreider RB, Kalman DS, Antonio J, et al. International Society of Sports Nutrition position stand: safety and efficacy of creatine supplementation in exercise, sport, and medicine. J Int Soc Sports Nutr 2017;14:18.
35. Branch JD. Effect of creatine supplementation on body composition and performance: a meta-analysis. Int J Sport Nutr Exerc Metab 2003;13(2):198–226.
36. Lanhers C, Pereira B, Naughton G, et al. Creatine supplementation and upper limb strength performance: a systematic review and meta-analysis. Sports Med 2017;47(1):163–73.
37. Schilling BK, Stone MH, Utter A, et al. Creatine supplementation and health variables: a retrospective study. Med Sci Sports Exerc 2001;33(2):183–8.
38. Dalbo VJ, Roberts MD, Stout JR, et al. Putting to rest the myth of creatine supplementation leading to muscle cramps and dehydration. Br J Sports Med 2008; 42(7):567–73.
39. Lancha Junior AH, Painelli VeS, Saunders B, et al. Nutritional strategies to modulate intracellular and extracellular buffering capacity during high-intensity exercise. Sports Med 2015;45(Suppl 1):S71–81.
40. Saunders B, Elliott-Sale K, Artioli GG, et al. β-alanine supplementation to improve exercise capacity and performance: a systematic review and meta-analysis. Br J Sports Med 2017;51(8):658–69.
41. Chung W, Shaw G, Anderson ME, et al. Effect of 10 week beta-alanine supplementation on competition and training performance in elite swimmers. Nutrients 2012;4(10):1441–53.
42. Bailey SJ, Varnham RL, DiMenna FJ, et al. Inorganic nitrate supplementation improves muscle oxygenation, O_2 uptake kinetics, and exercise tolerance at high but not low pedal rates. J Appl Physiol (1985) 2015;118(11):1396–405.
43. Thompson C, Wylie LJ, Fulford J, et al. Dietary nitrate improves sprint performance and cognitive function during prolonged intermittent exercise. Eur J Appl Physiol 2015;115(9):1825–34.
44. Wylie LJ, Ortiz de Zevallos J, Isidore T, et al. Dose-dependent effects of dietary nitrate on the oxygen cost of moderate-intensity exercise: acute vs. chronic supplementation. Nitric Oxide 2016;57:30–9.
45. Wylie LJ, Kelly J, Bailey SJ, et al. Beetroot juice and exercise: pharmacodynamic and dose-response relationships. J Appl Physiol (1985) 2013;115(3):325–36.
46. Hoon MW, Hopkins WG, Jones AM, et al. Nitrate supplementation and high-intensity performance in competitive cyclists. Appl Physiol Nutr Metab 2014; 39(9):1043–9.
47. Wylie LJ, Bailey SJ, Kelly J, et al. Influence of beetroot juice supplementation on intermittent exercise performance. Eur J Appl Physiol 2016;116(2):415–25.
48. Habermeyer M, Roth A, Guth S, et al. Nitrate and nitrite in the diet: how to assess their benefit and risk for human health. Mol Nutr Food Res 2015;59(1):106–28.
49. NSF International certified for sport. 2010. Available at: http://www.nsfsport.com/index.php. Accessed December 19, 2018.

50. The gold standard. Banned substances control group. 2018. Available at: https://www.bscg.org/. Accessed December 19, 2018.
51. USP dietary supplements and herbal medicines. Available at: https://www.usp.org/dietary-supplements-herbal-medicines. Accessed December 19, 2018.
52. Trusted by sport. 1999. Available at: Informed-Choice.org; https://www.informed-choice.org/about. Accessed December 19, 2018.
53. TRC. Natural standard. Sports medicine. 2018. Available at: https://naturalmedicines.therapeuticresearch.com/databases/sports-medicine.aspx. Accessed December 19, 2018.
54. Available at: ConsumerLab.com; https://www.consumerlab.com/results/. Accessed December 19, 2018.
55. U.S. Anti-Doping Agency. Supplement411. Realize. Recognize. Reduce. 2014. Available at: https://www.usada.org/substances/supplement-411/. Accessed December 19, 2018.
56. U.S. Food and Drug Administration. Dietary supplements. 2017. Available at: https://www.fda.gov/ForConsumers/ConsumerUpdates/ucm153239.htm. Accessed December 19, 2018.

Common Prescription Medications Used in Athletes

Benjamin Ferry, MD[a], Alexei DeCastro, MD[b], Scott Bragg, PharmD[c],*

KEYWORDS

- Athletes • Sports medicine • Medication use • Analgesics • Antibiotics
- Antihypertensives • Insulin • Therapeutic use exemptions

KEY POINTS

- Nonsteroidal anti-inflammatories have significant side effects and limited research in athletes and therefore should be used for the shortest possible duration in response to injuries. Acetaminophen is a relatively safe alternative analgesic.
- Inhaled β_2-agonists and corticosteroids remain the mainstay of asthma and exercise-induced respiratory disorders, and intranasal corticosteroids are the first-line option for allergic and nonallergic rhinitis in athletes.
- Athletes with diabetes require adjustments to their insulin regimen when participating in physical activity to minimize the risks of hypoglycemia and hyperglycemia.
- Angiotensin-converting enzyme inhibitors, angiotensin receptor blockers, and calcium-channel blockers are safe, effective options for the treatment of hypertension in athletes.
- Owing to the risk of QT prolongation and tendon rupture, the use of fluoroquinolones should generally be avoided in athletes.

INTRODUCTION

Although a generally young and healthy population, athletes' use of medications is not uncommon. In a 2009 study, 44% of track and field athletes of various ages and nationalities reported use of at least 1 medication.[1] From 2002 to 2014, nearly 70% of the participants in the men's FIFA World Cup used a medication at some point during the tournament.[2] The type and role of the medicines used is varied; some medications,

[a] Trident/MUSC Family Medicine Residency Program, Department of Family Medicine, Medical University of South Carolina, 9228 Medical Plaza Drive, Charleston, SC 29406, USA; [b] Department of Family Medicine, Medical University of South Carolina, College of Medicine, 9228 Medical Plaza Drive, Charleston, SC 29406, USA; [c] Department of Family Medicine, College of Medicine, College of Pharmacy, Clinical Pharmacy and Outcomes Sciences, Medical University of South Carolina, 280 Calhoun Street MSC 140, Charleston, SC 29425, USA
* Corresponding author.
E-mail address: braggsc@musc.edu

Prim Care Clin Office Pract 47 (2020) 49–64
https://doi.org/10.1016/j.pop.2019.10.003
0095-4543/20/© 2019 Elsevier Inc. All rights reserved.
primarycare.theclinics.com

such as nonsteroidal anti-inflammatories (NSAIDs) or acetaminophen, are aimed primarily at short-term symptom relief; others, such as inhaled β_2-agonists or insulin, are required for management of chronic conditions. A 2013 survey of US college students found that nearly 40% of students participating in "pick-up sports" used prescription medications in an attempt to enhance athletic performance.[3] Large-scale epidemiologic data about frequency of medication use is limited, particularly in the "weekend warrior" patient population. A 2006 study by Alaranta and colleagues[4] found that elite Finnish athletes were prescribed multiple medications, specifically NSAIDs, antibiotics, antiasthmatic and antiallergic medications, at a significantly higher rate than the general population. Despite the relative frequency at which these drugs are used, unique challenges and considerations exist when managing medications in an athlete. Attention must be paid to a medication's short- and long-term safety, effectiveness on achieving desired treatment outcomes, and effect on athletic performance, particularly in elite athletes. This article reviews the literature on common medications used by athletes and provides commentary on appropriate use.

ANALGESIC MEDICATIONS

NSAIDs are commonly used to help relieve pain, reduce inflammation, and hopefully enhance recovery in athletes of all levels.[4,5] It remains unclear, however, how safe NSAIDs are when used for musculoskeletal injuries and if use improves athletic performance. Inflammation is thought to be an important factor in cell and tissue regeneration, but it is theorized that if this process is frequently inhibited by medications such as NSAIDs, then muscle regeneration may be impaired.[6] In fact, some evidence has shown high-dose NSAID use may worsen muscle strength, protein synthesis, and hypertrophy after undergoing resistance training in young adults.[7,8] Fortunately, another study by Trappe and colleagues[9] in older athletes showed that ibuprofen 1200 mg daily and acetaminophen 4000 mg daily during 12 weeks of resistance training led to an increase in muscle mass and strength. Unfortunately, many risks exist with NSAIDs including acute kidney injury, hepatic impairment, bleeding, and cardiovascular events among others, which may warrant cautious use of NSAIDs in athletes.

All NSAIDs work to reduce pain and inflammation owing to inhibitory effects on the cyclooxygenase (COX) system, which is responsible for the production of prostaglandins and thromboxanes from arachidonic acid. NSAIDs are either nonselective inhibitors of both COX-1 and COX-2 (eg, ibuprofen, naproxen) or inhibit COX-2 selectively (eg, celecoxib). Inhibition of COX-2 is thought to be the primary pathway for reducing inflammation and pain, whereas inhibition of the COX-1 system causes several undesirable side effects such as bleeding, gastrointestinal ulcer formation, and kidney vasoconstriction.[10] When comparing the side effects of different NSAIDs, those that inhibit both COX-1 and COX-2 tend to cause higher rates of gastrointestinal bleeding and renal injury than those that inhibit COX-2 selectively.[11] All NSAIDs are linked with causing more cardiovascular events than nonuse, but selective COX-2 inhibitors are thought to pose a higher cardiovascular risk.[11,12]

When comparing the safety of various NSAIDs in athletes, no trial could be identified that reported the incidence of various adverse effects or if one NSAID was less risky than others. In the PRECISION trial, celecoxib was found to have a lower risk of gastrointestinal bleeding and renal injury compared with ibuprofen or naproxen without having a higher cardiovascular risk.[11] Clinicians have concern about the validity of this comparison, though, because the dose of celecoxib was limited to 100 mg twice daily, although 200 mg twice daily is commonly used in clinical practice. Naproxen is often thought to pose a lower risk of cardiovascular events than other

NSAIDs,[13] but not all trials have supported this finding.[11,12] Several trials have shown a higher cardiovascular risk with selective COX-2 inhibitors, requiring the removal of rofecoxib and valdecoxib from the US market. To minimize the risks posed by NSAIDs in athletes, they should be used at the lowest dose for the shortest period and should only be used in response to a musculoskeletal injury rather than to prevent pain before athletic activity.

Many questions remain unanswered when thinking about NSAID use in athletes. For example, do injectable NSAIDs pose higher or lower risks to athletes? Or is topical use associated with fewer risks and similar benefits to other NSAIDs? Ketorolac injections have become commonplace in professional and college athletes over the last 30 years since its US Food and Drug Administration approval. It remains the only injectable NSAID in the United States. When used as an intramuscular or intravenous injection, ketorolac has potent analgesic effects that have been shown to be similar to opiates such as morphine in multiple studies looking at postoperative pain relief and treatment of musculoskeletal injuries.[10] Ketorolac's safety concerns are similar to other NSAIDs, but it also is limited to a 5-day treatment course by the US Food and Drug Administration because it has a higher risk of gastrointestinal bleeding compared with other NSAIDs.

Topical NSAIDs are often deemed similarly effective with fewer systemic side effects when applied to localized pain. Diclofenac is the only topical NSAID approved in the United States and comes as a patch or gel. A recent Cochrane Review showed it was similarly effective for pain relief when compared with oral NSAIDs for acute sprains, strains, and overuse injuries. Topical NSAIDs only cause mild, transient skin reactions, which rarely causes treatment discontinuation, and have few reported systemic toxicities.[14] As a result, topical diclofenac should be a preferred option for localized pain if deemed clinically appropriate by a provider and if the more expensive topical product is financially feasible for the patient.

Acetaminophen is another medication commonly used in athletes to reduce pain, but unlike NSAIDs it is not thought to significantly contribute to anti-inflammatory effects. Some evidence exists, however, that acetaminophen may reduce protein synthesis or translational cell signaling after resistance exercise.[8,15] In contrast with NSAIDs, acetaminophen has more positive studies on improving endurance, performance, and muscle strength, so it might be considered before exercising to improve endurance or as a first-line option in patients who develop a musculoskeletal injury.[9,16–18]

Another potential benefit of acetaminophen in comparison to NSAIDs is its more favorable safety profile. Adverse events when taken at recommended doses are rare, although acetaminophen comes in multiple different combinations both over the counter and as a prescription so taking higher than recommended amounts (ie, >3 g/d without health care provider oversight or more than 4 g/d with provider oversight) is a common area of confusion with patients. Many patients may also claim that acetaminophen does not seem to help their pain when used on an as-needed basis. For this reason and for optimal pain control, athletes using acetaminophen for pain relief should take acetaminophen on a schedule of 650 mg every 6 hours or 1000 mg every 8 hours. **Table 1** provides an acute pain treatment review from the International Olympic Committee's (IOC) 2017 consensus statement.[19]

Prescribing of opiates in athletes is an area of debate considering many athletes report using opiates for nonmedical reasons after recovering from an injury and opiates have many serious risks (eg, respiratory depression, altered mental status, addiction).[20] In 2016, the Centers for Disease Control and Prevention published guidelines highlighting many concerns with using opiates in chronic noncancer pain and provided

Table 1
Medication management options for acute pain in athletes returning to play

Medication	Notes
Mild to moderate pain	
Oral acetaminophen	Loading dose up to 2 g, then 325–1000 mg every 4–6 h (max 4 g per 24 h)
Oral NSAIDs	Ibuprofen 400–800 mg every 4–6 h with food (max 3200 mg per 24 h) Naproxen 250–550 mg twice daily with food Ketorolac 10 mg every 4–6 h with food (max 40 mg per 24 h; only indicated short term [≤5 d]) Celecoxib 200–400 mg twice daily
Topical analgesics	Diclofenac patch (1.3%) topically twice daily to the most painful area; diclofenac gel (1.16%) topically 2–4 g 3–4 times daily to the affected area; diclofenac gel (2.32%) topically 2 g twice daily to affected area Rubefacient: methyl salicylate, turpentine oil Cooling sensation: menthol, camphor Vasodilation: histamine dihydrochloride, methyl nicotinate Irritation without rubefaction: capsaicin, capsicum oleoresin
Moderate to severe pain	
Injectable NSAIDs	Ketorolac 15–30 mg IM or IV up to 4 times a day at least 6 h apart or a single 60 mg injection

Medication options for acute pain management in athletes intending to return to play as organized by pain severity.

Abbreviations: IM, intramuscular; IV, intravenous.

Data from Hainline B, Derman W, Vernec A, et al. International Olympic Committee consensus statement on pain management in elite athletes. Br J Sports Med. 2017;51:1245–1258; and Wolters Kluwer Clinical Drug Information, Inc. (Lexi-Drugs). Wolters Kluwer Clinical Drug Information, Inc.; February 28, 2019.

recommendations to help decrease the risk of overdose and addiction. One of the practice-changing recommendations from these guidelines was that if opiates were chosen for treatment of acute pain a duration not exceeding 3 to 5 days was endorsed.[21] Opiates remain effective for treating short-term musculoskeletal injury pain in athletes, but considering the risks and lack of superior evidence of benefit, they should be used last line. Long-term use should be highly discouraged owing to a lack of long-term effectiveness data and serious safety concerns.

ALLERGIC RHINITIS AND ASTHMA MEDICATIONS

Physical activity can serve as a trigger for asthma, exercise-induced bronchoconstriction (EIB), and exercise-induced rhinitis. EIB is a narrowing of the airways that may occur with or without asthma. Symptoms of asthma and EIB include coughing, wheezing, or dyspnea.[22] For those with a diagnosis of asthma, exercise may trigger a significant exacerbation so clinicians and athletes should be mindful of how an athlete responds to different types of physical activity.[23] Exercise-induced rhinitis is one of the least known respiratory complications from physical activity and is characterized by sneezing, rhinorrhea, or nasal congestion.[23,24] Etiologies other than exercise for rhinitis or asthma exacerbations, such as environmental allergens, chemicals, or infection, are important to consider as well when discussing symptom control with patients.[25] For example, outdoor competitions or chlorine-treated pools may trigger symptoms that could be prevented with thoughtful planning. Regardless of the etiology, multiple medications exist for control of these conditions and are discussed in the next sections and **Table 2**.

Treatment Options for Asthma and Exercise-Induce Bronchospasm

Management of asthma and EIB involves use of several classes of inhaled bronchodilators. Short-acting β_2-agonists (SABAs), such as albuterol, are the preferred treatment of acute bronchospasm before, during, or after physical activity.[26] Albuterol is maximally effective within minutes of inhalation, but its effects only last for a few hours. Exercise produces a transient increase in airway reactivity, which can be managed prophylactically with SABA inhalation 30 minutes before initiation of activity. However, in a 2011 survey, fewer than 25% of pediatric patients with asthma used a SABA

Table 2
Medication options for managing asthma and allergic rhinitis in athletes

Condition	Medication Class	Generic Examples	Considerations
Asthma/EIB	Short acting β_2-Agonist	Albuterol Salbutamol Levalbuterol	Rescue inhaler for EIB symptoms Prophylaxis before exercise Likely needs TUE
	Long acting β_2-Agonist	Formoterol Salmeterol	Prophylaxis for EIB Not for acute bronchospasm Not monotherapy for maintenance Adjunct to ICS for maintenance therapy Likely needs TUE
	ICS	Fluticasone Budesonide Beclomethasone	First line for asthma maintenance No usefulness in rescue therapy or EIB prophylaxis
Allergic rhinitis	Intranasal corticosteroids	Fluticasone Budesonide Beclomethasone Mometasone Triamcinolone	First line option Effect starting within 12 h, maximally effective after a few days Likely no TUE required Minimal side effects
	Antihistamines	Loratadine Cetirizine Azelastine (IN) Olopatadine (IN)	Second-generation agents are preferred Possible adjunct to intranasal corticosteroids Avoid first-generation options owing to sedation
	Leukotriene modifiers	Montelukast Zafirlukast	Potential adjunct option for AR, asthma, EIB Can improve performance for asthmatic athletes
	Decongestants	Phenylephrine Pseudoephedrine Oxymetazoline (IN)	Short-term (3–5 d) use only Effective for nasal congestion/ obstruction Significant side effects

Abbreviations: AR, allergic rhinitis; EIB, exercise-induce bronchospasm; ICS, inhaled corticosteroid; IN, intranasal; TUE, therapeutic use exemption.
Data from Refs.[22,26,36,44]

before exercise always or most of the time.[27] Counseling on appropriate use of pre-exercise prophylaxis to reduce EIB should be provided to athletes as a result.

Long-term management and control of asthma is generally the same as in nonath-letes. The 2018 Global Initiative for Asthma guidelines identify inhaled corticosteroids (ICS) as the first-line option for long-term maintenance therapy.[26] Frequent symptoms with exercise may represent the need for escalation of maintenance therapy, which may include either an increase of the ICS dose or adding a long-acting inhaled β_2-agonist (LABA) to the current regimen.[26] Although increasing the dose of the ICS is an option, adding a LABA to an ICS is likely more effective at decreasing the risk of an asthma exacerbation.[28] Fortunately, there is evidence that an ICS may have a non–dose-dependent protective effective against symptoms of EIB.[29] Although they should not be used as long-term monotherapy for asthma, LABAs such as salmeterol and formoterol can also be used prophylactically for control of exercise-induced symptoms. Time to effect onset of formoterol is similar to SABAs; however, LABAs are not recommended for relief of acute bronchospasm.[26] Tachyphylaxis results with frequent use of LABAs as seen in the decreases in duration of effect from 12 hours to 5 hours with overuse.[22]

The National Athletic Trainers' Association recommends that each patient with asthma should have a rescue inhaler on hand for all practices and games, and the ath-letic trainer should also ideally have a back-up inhaler on hand for each athlete.[30] Use of a spacer with any use of a metered-dose inhaler is encouraged to improve effectiveness.[26]

Although there is concern about theoretic performance enhancement with the use of inhaled β_2-agonists, multiple studies have demonstrated no improvement in exer-cise performance in nonasthmatic athletes.[31–33] Regardless, β_2-agonist use in colle-giate and elite athletes remains restricted. β_2-Agonists are on the most recent list of substances banned by the National Collegiate Athletic Association (NCAA) and the World Anti-Doping Agency (WADA).[34,35] For athletes needing a therapeutic use exemption (TUE) to use β_2-agonists for asthma, specific limits are set for each agent to minimize the potential for overuse. Thresholds for urine levels of salbutamol and for-moterol to detect use beyond therapeutic purposes are used by WADA. Providers should reference the WADA, NCAA, IOC, or other relevant web sites for the most up-to-date policies on medication restrictions.

Treatment Options for Exercise-Induced Rhinitis

Intranasal corticosteroids are the first-line option for athletes dealing with rhinitis symptoms and can be used either alone or together with oral antihistamines.[36] The use of intranasal corticosteroids has been shown to be safe and effective for control-ling symptoms with allergic and nonallergic rhinitis.[22] Intranasal corticosteroids may improve sleep quality and daytime fatigue in athletes, which are important factors for optimal recovery from training and rest for competition.[37] Side effects, such as nasal bleeding, may occur in the nares but are typically mild.[24] Unlike systemic corti-costeroids, inhaled and intranasal corticosteroids are not included on the list of pro-hibited medications from WADA.[35]

Oral systemic antihistamines are also considered a first-line alternative for allergic rhinitis and nonallergic rhinitis.[25,36] The main side effect of first-generation antihista-mines is sedation, which can impair reaction time and performance, but this side effect is minimal with the second-generation agents (eg, cetirizine, fexofenadine).[25,36] Intra-nasal antihistamines (eg, azelastine, olopatadine) are an alternative to oral antihista-mines, which may also limit sedation seen with oral options. A combination product of an intranasal corticosteroid and antihistamine (ie, azelastine and fluticasone) is also available, and it has shown to be more effective at improving moderate to severe symptoms of seasonal allergic rhinitis than either agent alone.[38] Although aerobic and endurance activities seem to generate a histamine release in skeletal muscles as part of a fundamental exercise response,[39,40] research on the impact of antihistamines on athletic performance is limited.[41]

Montelukast is an anti-inflammatory agent that works as an antagonist of type 1 cysteinyl-leukotriene receptors, helping to prevent allergen-induced airway inflammation.[42] Evidence supports its use in the management of asthma, EIB, and allergic rhinitis.[42] Studies suggest that montelukast can improve exercise performance for athletes with asthma or EIB,[43,44] but it was not found to be beneficial for nonasthmatic endurance athletes.[45]

Oral and intranasal decongestants are second-line options for the short-term management of nasal congestion.[24] The risk of rebound congestion exists with prolonged use (ie, >3–5 days), but this risk may be minimized by concomitant intranasal corticosteroids.[46] The NCAA and WADA have differing restrictions on oral decongestants, although use of phenylephrine and pseudoephedrine is permissible under both organizations so long as pseudoephedrine is not present in supratherapeutic amounts in urine drug testing.[34,35] Intranasal decongestants have less pronounced side effects and more immediate onset of action than their oral counterparts, but have little effect on nasal itching, sneezing, or rhinorrhea. Side effects more commonly seen with oral decongestants include irritability, dizziness, headache, insomnia, tremor, palpitations, and urinary retention.[24]

ANTIBIOTICS

It has been reported that athletes are prescribed oral antibiotics at almost twice the rate as the general population with the intent of returning athletes to play sooner.[6] All antibiotics have potential adverse effects with use, but in athletes particular attention should be placed on antibiotics with the potential for corrected QT (QTc) interval prolongation, tendon injury, nerve damage, glycemic fluctuation, and aortic dissection. Fluoroquinolones of note can cause all of these adverse effects so use in an athlete should be cautioned despite recent expanded use of fluoroquinolones in community-acquired pneumonia and sinusitis.

Prolongation of the QT interval is one of the most critical adverse effects associated with the use of fluoroquinolones, although the overall risk of torsades de pointes is low.[47] Fluoroquinolones prolong the QT interval by blocking voltage-gated potassium channels. Of the different fluoroquinolone options, moxifloxacin carries the greatest risk of QTc prolongation and ciprofloxacin has the lowest risk for QTc prolongation and the lowest rate of torsades. Other antibiotics with known QTc prolongation include macrolide antibiotics (eg, azithromycin, clarithromycin) and trimethoprim/sulfamethoxazole.[48,49] Regardless of the specific antibiotic used, providers should exercise caution prescribing antibiotics to an athlete with predisposing risk factors for torsades de pointes such as long QT syndrome. Athletes with known long QT syndrome may be able to participate in competitive sports,[48] but any QTc-prolonging medications should be strictly avoided in this population. Additionally, prescribing multiple medications associated with QT interval prolongation should be cautioned in all patients.

Tendinopathy and tendon rupture have also been reported in athletes with use of most fluoroquinolones, but the overall incidence is low. The Achilles tendon is the most commonly affected site, but injury has also been reported to occur in the rotator cuff, hand, biceps, thumb, and other sites.[50] The reported mechanism of injury is free radical accumulation in the central avascular portion of the Achilles tendon (ie, watershed area) during the inflammatory process.[51] Despite a low incidence of tendon injury associated with fluoroquinolone use in athletes, their use should be limited because the injury is so significant. Ciprofloxacin is the most often associated with tendon injury, although increased injury risk has been reported with the use of other fluoroquinolones as well. The median duration of treatment before the onset of tendon injury is 8 days, but symptoms may occur as early as 2 hours after the first dose and as late as 6 months after discontinuing treatment.[50] Patients over the age of 60 who used corticosteroids are at the highest risk of developing Achilles tendinopathy or rupture as compared with the general population.[52] Other reported risk factors for tendon rupture with fluoroquinolone use include chronic kidney disease, end-stage renal disease, or receiving a kidney transplant.

Another more recent warning with fluoroquinolone use is the potential increased risk of aortic aneurysm and dissection. Athletes with known aortic aneurysm or increased risk of dissection should avoid using fluoroquinolones. Other risk factors for aortic dissection include Marfan syndrome, Ehlers-Danlos syndrome, peripheral atherosclerosis, and hypertension.[53]

DIABETES MEDICATIONS

The management of diabetes in athletes often involves the treatment of patients diagnosed with type 1 diabetes mellitus because athletes tend to be more physically active and younger, 2 protective factors against developing insulin resistance.[54,55] As a result, this section is geared toward the treatment of athletes with type 1 diabetes, but many of the strategies can also be applied to athletes with insulin-dependent type 2 diabetes. Athletes with uncomplicated type 1 diabetes are capable of the same level of physical performance and exercise capacity as individuals without type 1 diabetes.[54] Exercise is a key component of diabetes management and is associated with positive effects on glucose control, cardiovascular events, mortality, and quality of life.[56] Providers must account for the type, duration, and intensity of exercise that an athlete will be participating in when creating an insulin regimen and revising that regimen after monitoring for adverse effects. The overall goals with insulin management around exercise are avoiding exercise-induced hypoglycemia, preventing hyperglycemia and ketosis, and ensuring optimal performance.[55]

Physical activity leads to a complex balance of multiple processes to maintain euglycemia, including increases in peripheral glucose uptake, glucagon secretion, hepatic glycogenolysis and gluconeogenesis, and lipid lipolysis. In addition, there are counterregulatory responses involving the release of growth hormone, cortisol, and epinephrine.[57,58] These changes provide adequate energy stores to maintain longer periods of peak physical performance and then prepares an athlete for future physical activity. This recovery phase may last between 24 and 72 hours after exercise.[56] In type 1 diabetes, the body is not able to alter exogenously administered insulin as an athlete without diabetes might to maintain euglycemia in the setting of these additional responses. Participation in sports has many logistical challenges (eg, few breaks, various levels of intensity, inability to readily monitor blood glucose) as well, which may impact management. Care of an athlete with diabetes requires an individualized, multifaceted approach, including blood glucose monitoring, carbohydrate consumption, and adjustment of insulin doses.[55,58,59]

An athlete should plan on consuming additional carbohydrates if exercising unexpectedly and unable to adjust their insulin regimen beforehand or if participating in prolonged exercise (ie, >1 hour).[58] Carbohydrates should also be consumed before the initiation of exercise if blood glucose is less than 100 mg/dL, if at any point a patient were to have a true low during exercise (ie, blood glucose <70 mg/dL), and shortly after conclusion of exercise.[59] **Table 3** provides specific recommendations to consider regarding carbohydrate intake around exercise.

Table 3 Diabetes management treatment strategies for athletes on insulin	
Treatment Considerations	**Adjustment Strategies**
Carbohydrate intake	
Increase carbohydrate intake around exercise	Eat 30–60 g of carbohydrates before prolonged exercise (ie, >1 h per session); consider increased carbohydrate consumption for intense exercise if durations of exercise are shorter
	Additional carbohydrates in excess of 60 g may be required depending on an athlete's response to activity and its duration
	If blood glucose is <100 mg/dL before exercise, eat before activity
	If blood glucose falls low during exercise, the activity should be stopped, the blood glucose should be appropriately treated with 15–30 g of fast-acting glucose, this should be repeated after 15 min if still low, and once >70 mg/dL a complex carbohydrate snack should be given to keep the blood sugar up during further exercise
	After each exercise session, a snack should be eaten within 30 min of stopping exercise
Blood glucose monitoring	
Increase frequency of blood glucose checks	Test blood glucose before meals and with 2-h postprandial checks
	Check blood glucose before, during, and after periods of physical activity
	If having long durations of exercise, consider checking every 30 min
	Contemplate assessing overnight glucose values if having more intense activity, longer durations of exercise, recent start of a new training regimen, or a history of severe hypoglycemic events
Insulin adjustments	
Changes in insulin absorption	More rapid absorption of insulin if exercise begins <30 min after injection
	Heat (eg, saunas, showers) applied to an insulin injection site can speed insulin absorption
	Cold (eg, ice, cool towels, cold spray) applied to an insulin injection site can slow insulin absorption
	Extreme outdoor temperatures (ie, <36°F or >86°F) can decrease insulin efficacy
Insulin pump dosing	Reduce basal insulin rate 1–2 h before exercise by 20%–50%
	Consider continued 20% reduction in basal rate after exercise for 24–72 h
	Reduce insulin bolus by 50% at meal before exercise
	Reduce evening meal bolus by 50% if concern for nighttime hypoglycemia
Multiple-daily injection dosing	Reduce insulin bolus by 50% at meal before exercise
	Reduce evening meal bolus by 50% if concern for nighttime hypoglycemia

Note: Bolus adjustments recommended with the assumption that exercise is within 2 h of bolus administration.
Data from Refs.[26,58,59]

Frequent blood glucose monitoring is important in titration of insulin for an athlete and prevention of low or high blood glucose. In a 2005 article, Hornsby and Chetlin[55] recommend testing before and after meals; before, during, and after exercise; and overnight if concerned about hypoglycemia. Monitoring glucose more frequently (ie, every 30 minutes) during extended activity and after exercise (ie, every 2–4 hours) is recommended considering the many factors on blood glucose homeostasis and the phases of physiologic effects that occur around exercise.[59] A 2007 study by McMahon and colleagues[60] suggested that there may be a biphasic increase in insulin sensitivity after afternoon exercise, with increased sensitivity occurring immediately after exercise and again 7 to 11 hours after exercise, emphasizing the importance of incorporating evening and nighttime glucose checks. For a summary of typical blood glucose monitoring recommendations, see **Table 3**. One exciting option for many athletes with diabetes is using a continuous glucose monitor, which may help to identify periods of hypoglycemia or hyperglycemia without an increased burden of capillary glucose checks. The drawback of this technology is it typically lags capillary glucose values by 10 to 20 minutes because it tests interstitial fluid glucose measurements, so it will not completely eliminate the need for some blood glucose testing.[57]

Although the American Diabetes Association proposes a trial and error approach to the management of insulin during exercise, the National Athletic Trainers' Association put forth a 2007 position statement with recommendations for insulin management around periods of physical activity that can serve as a starting point for most athletes. Insulin dose reduction strategies are tailored to patients on an insulin pump or multiple daily injections.[59] A summary of these recommendations is included in **Table 3**. Continuation of a patient's standard mealtime dose with subsequent exercise is associated with a higher risk of hypoglycemia regardless of exercise intensity,[61] necessitating empiric insulin dose reductions for anticipated physical activity. Adjustments to the recommendations in **Table 3** should be made based on the anticipated intensity, duration of exercise, response to previous activity of similar intensity and duration, and goals of the patient. Larger empiric reductions should be expected for more intense exercise and longer durations of activity.[61]

Although low blood glucose is the most feared concern with athletes on insulin, exercise-induced hyperglycemia is another phenomenon that providers and patients should try to minimize. Athletes receiving continuous subcutaneous insulin infusion with an insulin pump may be at reduced risk for postexercise hyperglycemia without increasing the risk for hypoglycemia when compared with multiple daily injections.[62] Thankfully, an insulin pump offers great flexibility with insulin delivery making it a preferred option for insulin dose adjustments with exercise.

ANTIHYPERTENSIVES

Health care providers should be familiar with recommendations for completing a preparticipation examination to identify athletes in need of extra monitoring for cardiovascular disease and those in need of treatment for hypertension. This screening opportunity may help to identify individuals who are at high risk of sudden cardiac death and reduce the risk of complications imposed by hypertension in athletes.[63] Thoughtful prescribing of antihypertensives in athletes includes multiple factors such as compelling medical indications, adverse effects seen with antihypertensives, and knowing the sport in which an athlete competes.

Unfortunately, antihypertensive medications are commonly needed in athletes despite the blood pressure-lowering effects seen with regular exercise. Many demographic factors may increase the likelihood that an athlete develops hypertension. **Table 4** presents several risk factors highlighted in previous literature.[63,64] Lifestyle modifications such as weight loss, dietary salt restriction, and moderation of alcohol intake are recommended as first-line treatment for athletes with uncontrolled blood pressure.[65] If medication therapy is required as an adjunct to lifestyle modifications in an athlete, angiotensin-converting enzyme inhibitors, angiotensin II receptor blockers, or dihydropyridine calcium channel blockers are recommended. These classes of medication are preferred in athletes because they have fewer side effects, do not inhibit exercise capacity, and are not problematic from a banned substance perspective.[63] When choosing between these options, treatment providers should consider specific medical indications for various antihypertensives and ethnic response to different medications. As an example, African American patients typically respond better to calcium channel blockers instead of angiotensin-converting enzyme inhibitors or angiotensin II receptor blockers. In athletes with diabetes mellitus or chronic kidney disease, an angiotensin-converting enzyme inhibitor or angiotensin II receptor blocker should be preferred considering their nephroprotective effects.

Several concerns exist with other classes of antihypertensive drugs. Thiazide diuretics are typically one of the first-line options for the treatment of hypertension, but in athletes there are concerns that they could impair strength and endurance via dehydration and lead to more electrolyte disturbances, such as hypokalemia and hypomagnesemia. Diuretics are also a banned substance in many sports because they can be used to mask performance-enhancing drugs by increasing urinary elimination.[64,65] In recent years, beta-blockers have become much less preferred for hypertension unless having a specific indication such as an arrhythmia, myocardial infarction, or congestive heart failure. These agents should rarely be used in athletes because they can impair exercise capacity. They also may be a banned substance in shooting and precision sports, where they could be taken to gain a competitive advantage.[65] Other antihypertensives such as aldosterone antagonists, alpha-2 agonists, alpha blockers, and direct vasodilators are associated with more side effects and have less evidence of benefit on patient-oriented outcomes, so they should be used sparingly in athletes.

Table 4
Risk factors for developing hypertension in athletes

Lifestyle Parameters	Comorbidities	Other Patient Demographics
High dietary salt intake	Diabetes mellitus	Male sex
Smoking or chewing tobacco	Obesity	African American race
Excessive alcohol intake	Anxiety disorders	Family history of
Caffeine intake	Hyperthyroidism	hypertension
Medication use (eg, ESAs, NSAIDs, anabolic steroids, stimulant use, HGH, illicit drug use)	Renal disease (eg, CKD, congenital abnormalities, nephrotic syndrome, PCKD, parenchymal disease)	High stress levels

Risk factors for hypertension in athletes divided by the categories: lifestyle parameters, comorbidities, and other patient demographics.

Abbreviations: CKD, chronic kidney disease; ESAs, erythropoietin-stimulating agents; HGH, human growth hormone; NSAIDs, nonsteroidal anti-inflammatory drugs; PCDK, polycystic kidney disease.

Data from Niedfeldt MW. Managing hypertension in athletes and physically active patients. Am Fam Physician. 2002;66(3):445–453; and Pelto H. Hypertensive medications in competitive athletes. Curr Sports Med Rep. 2017;16(1):45–49.

THERAPEUTIC USE EXEMPTIONS

In athletes diagnosed with a condition that requires the use of a drug prohibited by their sports' governing body, they may be given a TUE to allow use of the medication. Elite athletes have been reported to use supplements or medications for performance enhancement with or without physician consultation.[66] The TUE process is designed to balance athletes' use of needed medications while promoting a level playing field by ensuring athletes are not misusing medications in an attempt to boost performance.

Certain substances are completely prohibited in sports per WADA, IOC, NCAA, and US Anti-doping Agency guidelines, but there are substances that are allowed if the concentration is below a threshold level. There are also medications that could be considered doping agents that may be allowed for medical treatment, such as β_2-agonists and corticosteroids. Governing bodies may make exceptions for in-competition versus out-of-competition use of certain medications as well, which may impact the need for a TUE. For example, as previously discussed, there is no evidence of performance enhancement with β_2-agonist use in nonasthmatic athletes, but athletes still attempt to use the medication for such. In the 2000 Summer Olympic games in Sydney, Australia, a substantial increase was seen in athletes indicating they had asthma and needed treatment with a β_2-agonist compared with the previous 1996 Olympics. Most of this use was seen in triathletes and endurance athletes, but this led the IOC to randomly test more participants for doping.[67]

Prescribing medications in athletes must be a very deliberate process to ensure an athlete is in compliance with relevant antidoping guidelines. TUEs have strict criteria, so it is imperative that prescribing providers are aware of the requirements and procedures for applying for a TUE.

SUMMARY

The treatment of common conditions in athletes requires knowledge of the distinct considerations relevant to this population. Prescribers must balance the safety, efficacy, performance impact, and regulatory restrictions of each medication when creating a treatment plan. Continued research on the safety and effectiveness of drugs in athletes of all levels is needed moving forward to better educate clinicians and athletes on optimal medication use strategies.

DISCLOSURE

The authors of this article have no financial relationships or affiliations to disclose.

REFERENCES

1. Tscholl P, Alonso JM, Dollé G, et al. The use of drugs and nutritional supplements in top-level track and field athletes. Am J Sports Med 2010;38(1):133–40.
2. Tscholl PM, Vaso M, Weber A, et al. High prevalence of medication use in professional football tournaments including the World Cups between 2002 and 2014: a narrative review with a focus on NSAIDs. Br J Sports Med 2015;49(9):580–2.
3. Hoyte CO, Albert D, Heard KJ. The use of energy drinks, dietary supplements, and prescription medications by United States college students to enhance athletic performance. J Community Health 2013;38(3):575–80.
4. Alaranta A, Alaranta H, Heliövaara M, et al. Ample use of physician-prescribed medications in Finnish elite athletes. Int J Sports Med 2006;27(11):919–25.
5. Harle CA, Danielson EC, Derman W, et al. Analgesic management of pain in elite athletes: a systematic review. Clin J Sport Med 2018;28(5):417–26.

6. Alaranta A, Alaranta H, Helenius I. Use of prescription drugs in athletes. Sports Med 2008;38(6):449–63.
7. Lilja M, Mandic M, Apro W, et al. High doses of anti-inflammatory drugs compromise muscle strength and hypertrophic adaptations to resistance training in young adults. Acta Physiol 2018;222(2):e12948.
8. Trappe TA, White F, Lambert CP, et al. Effect of ibuprofen and acetaminophen on postexercise muscle protein synthesis. Am J Physiol Endocrinol Metab 2002; 282(3):E551–6.
9. Trappe TA, Carroll CC, Dickinson JM, et al. Influence of acetaminophen and ibuprofen on skeletal muscle adaptations to resistance exercise in older adults. Am J Physiol Regul Integr Comp Physiol 2011;300(3):R655–62.
10. Matava MJ. Injectable nonsteroidal anti-inflammatory drugs in sport. Clin J Sport Med 2018;28(5):443–50.
11. Nissen SE, Yeomans ND, Solomon DH, et al. Cardiovascular safety of celecoxib, naproxen, or ibuprofen for arthritis. N Engl J Med 2016;375(26):2519–29.
12. Bally M, Dendukuri N, Rich B, et al. Risk of acute myocardial infarction with NSAIDs in real world use: Bayesian meta-analysis of individual patient data. BMJ 2017;357:j1909.
13. Bhala N, Emberson J, Merhi A, et al. Vascular and upper gastrointestinal effects of non-steroidal anti-inflammatory drugs: meta-analyses of individual participant data from randomised trials. Lancet 2013;382(9894):769–79.
14. Derry S, Moore RA, Gaskell H, et al. Topical NSAIDs for acute musculoskeletal pain in adults. Cochrane Database Syst Rev 2015;(6):CD007402.
15. D'Lugos AC, Patel SH, Ormsby JC, et al. Prior acetaminophen consumption impacts the early adaptive cellular response of human skeletal muscle to resistance exercise. J Appl Physiol 2018;124(4):1012–24.
16. Foster J, Taylor L, Chrismas BC, et al. The influence of acetaminophen on repeated sprint cycling performance. Eur J Appl Physiol 2014;114(1):41–8.
17. Mauger AR, Jones AM, Williams CA. Influence of acetaminophen on performance during time trial cycling. J Appl Physiol 2010;108(1):98–104.
18. Mauger AR, Taylor L, Harding C, et al. Acute acetaminophen (paracetamol) ingestion improves time to exhaustion during exercise in the heat. Exp Physiol 2014;99(1):164–71.
19. Hainline B, Derman W, Vernec A, et al. International Olympic Committee consensus statement on pain management in elite athletes. Br J Sports Med 2017;51(17):1245–58.
20. Ford JA, Pomykacz C, Veliz P, et al. Sports involvement, injury history, and non-medical use of prescription opioids among college students: an analysis with a national sample. Am J Addict 2018;27(1):15–22.
21. Dowell D, Haegerich TM, Chou R. CDC Guideline for Prescribing Opioids for Chronic Pain - United States, 2016. MMWR Recomm Rep 2016;65(1):1–52.
22. Schwartz LB, Delgado L, Craig T, et al. Exercise-induced hypersensitivity syndromes in recreational and competitive athletes: a PRACTALL consensus report (what the general practitioner should know about sports and allergy). Allergy 2008;63(8):953–61.
23. Bacharier LB, Boner A, Carlsen KH, et al. Diagnosis and treatment of asthma in childhood: a PRACTALL consensus report. Allergy 2008;63(1):5–34.
24. Bousquet J, Khaltaev N, Cruz AA, et al. Allergic Rhinitis and its Impact on Asthma (ARIA) 2008 update (in collaboration with the World Health Organization, GA(2) LEN and AllerGen). Allergy 2008;63(86):8–160.

25. Steelant B, Hox V, Hellings PW, et al. Exercise and sinonasal disease. Immunol Allergy Clin North Am 2018;38(2):259–69.
26. Asthma GIf. Global strategy for asthma management and prevention, 2018. 2018. Available at: www.ginasthma.org. Accessed April 22, 2019.
27. Ostrom NK, Eid NS, Craig TJ, et al. Exercise-induced bronchospasm in children with asthma in the United States: results from the Exercise-Induced Bronchospasm Landmark Survey. Allergy Asthma Proc 2011;32(6):425–30.
28. Sobieraj DM, Weeda ER, Nguyen E, et al. Association of inhaled corticosteroids and long-acting beta-agonists as controller and quick relief therapy with exacerbations and symptom control in persistent asthma: a systematic review and meta-analysis. JAMA 2018;319(14):1485–96.
29. Hofstra WB, Neijens HJ, Duiverman EJ, et al. Dose-responses over time to inhaled fluticasone propionate treatment of exercise- and methacholine-induced bronchoconstriction in children with asthma. Pediatr Pulmonol 2000;29(6):415–23.
30. Miller MG, Weiler JM, Baker R, et al. National Athletic Trainers' Association position statement: management of asthma in athletes. J Athl Train 2005;40(3):224–45.
31. Eckerström F, Rex CE, Maagaard M, et al. Exercise performance after salbutamol inhalation in non-asthmatic, non-athlete individuals: a randomised, controlled, cross-over trial. BMJ Open Sport Exerc Med 2018;4(1):e000397.
32. Kindermann W, Meyer T. Inhaled beta2 agonists and performance in competitive athletes. Br J Sports Med 2006;40(1):i43–7.
33. Kindermann W. Do inhaled beta(2)-agonists have an ergogenic potential in non-asthmatic competitive athletes? Sports Med 2007;37(2):95–102.
34. Association NCAA. 2018–19 NCAA banned drugs. NCAA Sports Science Institute. 2019. Available at: http://www.ncaa.org/sites/default/files/2018-19NCAA_Banned_Drugs_20180608.pdf. Accessed April 22, 2019.
35. Agency WA-D. Prohibited list. The World Anti-Doping Code International Standard. 2019. https://www.wada-ama.org/sites/default/files/wada_2019_english_prohibited_list.pdf. Accessed April 22, 2019.
36. Small P, Keith PK, Kim H. Allergic rhinitis. Allergy Asthma Clin Immunol 2018;14(2):51.
37. Hughes K, Glass C, Ripchinski M, et al. Efficacy of the topical nasal steroid budesonide on improving sleep and daytime somnolence in patients with perennial allergic rhinitis. Allergy 2003;58(5):380–5.
38. Hampel FC, Ratner PH, Van Bavel J, et al. Double-blind, placebo-controlled study of azelastine and fluticasone in a single nasal spray delivery device. Ann Allergy Asthma Immunol 2010;105(2):168–73.
39. Luttrell MJ, Halliwill JR. The intriguing role of histamine in exercise responses. Exerc Sport Sci Rev 2017;45(1):16–23.
40. Romero SA, Hocker AD, Mangum JE, et al. Evidence of a broad histamine footprint on the human exercise transcriptome. J Physiol 2016;594(17):5009–23.
41. Montgomery LC, Deuster PA. Effects of antihistamine medications on exercise performance. Implications for sportspeople. Sports Med 1993;15(3):179–95.
42. Nayak A, Langdon RB. Montelukast in the treatment of allergic rhinitis: an evidence-based review. Drugs 2007;67(6):887–901.
43. Leff JA, Busse WW, Pearlman D, et al. Montelukast, a leukotriene-receptor antagonist, for the treatment of mild asthma and exercise-induced bronchoconstriction. N Engl J Med 1998;339(3):147–52.

44. Steinshamn S, Sandsund M, Sue-Chu M, et al. Effects of montelukast on physical performance and exercise economy in adult asthmatics with exercise-induced bronchoconstriction. Scand J Med Sci Sports 2002;12(4):211–7.
45. Sue-Chu M, Sandsund M, Holand B, et al. Montelukast does not affect exercise performance at subfreezing temperature in highly trained non-asthmatic endurance athletes. Int J Sports Med 2000;21(6):424–8.
46. Baroody FM, Brown D, Gavanescu L, et al. Oxymetazoline adds to the effectiveness of fluticasone furoate in the treatment of perennial allergic rhinitis. J Allergy Clin Immunol 2011;127(4):927–34.
47. Golzari H, Dawson NV, Speroff T, et al. Prolonged QTc intervals on admission electrocardiograms: prevalence and correspondence with admission electrolyte abnormalities. Conn Med 2007;71(7):389–97.
48. Fayock K, Voltz M, Sandella B, et al. Antibiotic precautions in athletes. Sports Health 2014;6(4):321–5.
49. Lopez JA, Harold JG, Rosenthal MC, et al. QT prolongation and torsades de pointes after administration of trimethoprim-sulfamethoxazole. Am J Cardiol 1987;59(4):376–7.
50. Khaliq Y, Zhanel GG. Fluoroquinolone-associated tendinopathy: a critical review of the literature. Clin Infect Dis 2003;36(11):1404–10.
51. Seeger JD, West WA, Fife D, et al. Achilles tendon rupture and its association with fluoroquinolone antibiotics and other potential risk factors in a managed care population. Pharmacoepidemiol Drug Saf 2006;15(11):784–92.
52. Wise BL, Peloquin C, Choi H, et al. Impact of age, sex, obesity, and steroid use on quinolone-associated tendon disorders. Am J Med 2012;125(12):1228.e23–8.
53. Daneman N, Lu H, Redelmeier DA. Fluoroquinolones and collagen associated severe adverse events: a longitudinal cohort study. BMJ Open 2015;5(11): e010077.
54. Horton WB, Subauste JS. Care of the athlete with type 1 diabetes mellitus: a clinical review. Int J Endocrinol Metab 2016;14(2):e36091.
55. Hornsby WG Jr, Chetlin RD. Management of competitive athletes with diabetes. Diabetes Spectrum 2005;18(2):102–7.
56. Colberg SR, Sigal RJ, Fernhall B, et al. Exercise and type 2 diabetes: the American College of Sports Medicine and the American Diabetes Association: joint position statement. Diabetes Care 2010;33(12):e147–67.
57. Codella R, Terruzzi I, Luzi L. Why should people with type 1 diabetes exercise regularly? Acta Diabetol 2017;54(7):615–30.
58. Gallen IW, Hume C, Lumb A. Fuelling the athlete with type 1 diabetes. Diabetes Obes Metab 2011;13(2):130–6.
59. Jimenez CC, Corcoran MH, Crawley JT, et al. National athletic trainers' association position statement: management of the athlete with type 1 diabetes mellitus. J Athl Train 2007;42(4):536–45.
60. McMahon SK, Ferreira LD, Ratnam N, et al. Glucose requirements to maintain euglycemia after moderate-intensity afternoon exercise in adolescents with type 1 diabetes are increased in a biphasic manner. J Clin Endocrinol Metab 2007; 92(3):963–8.
61. Rabasa-Lhoret R, Bourque J, Ducros F, et al. Guidelines for premeal insulin dose reduction for postprandial exercise of different intensities and durations in type 1 diabetic subjects treated intensively with a basal-bolus insulin regimen (ultralente-lispro). Diabetes Care 2001;24(4):625–30.
62. Yardley JE, Iscoe KE, Sigal RJ, et al. Insulin pump therapy is associated with less post-exercise hyperglycemia than multiple daily injections: an observational

study of physically active type 1 diabetes patients. Diabetes Technol Ther 2013; 15(1):84–8.

63. Pelto H. Hypertensive medications in competitive athletes. Curr Sports Med Rep 2017;16(1):45–9.

64. Niedfeldt MW. Managing hypertension in athletes and physically active patients. Am Fam Physician 2002;66(3):445–52.

65. Asplund C. Treatment of hypertension in athletes: an evidence-based review. Phys Sportsmed 2010;38(1):37–44.

66. Tsitsimpikou C, Tsiokanos A, Tsarouhas K, et al. Medication use by athletes at the Athens 2004 Summer Olympic Games. Clin J Sport Med 2009;19(1):33–8.

67. Thuyne WV, Delbeke FT. Declared use of medication in sports. Clin J Sport Med 2008;18(2):143–7.

Common Medical Concerns of the Female Athlete

Siobhan M. Statuta, MD[a,b],*, Colton L. Wood, MD[c], Lisa K. Rollins, PhD[d]

KEYWORDS

• Female • Athlete • Female athlete triad • Pregnancy • Iron

KEY POINTS

- When counseling a patient on initiating or continuing an exercise regimen during pregnancy, it is advised to follow a stepwise approach; start out slow and easy, ensure excellent nutrition, rest, and hydration.
- The female athlete triad is a complex condition that, if left unrecognized or untreated, can lead to serious and longstanding negative health outcomes. It is thus important to screen for this condition early.
- Patellofemoral pain is a common, multifactorial condition that often turns chronic. Exercise prescription is a helpful treatment modality and is often best addressed through a gym-based program.
- Anterior cruciate ligament injuries are more common in female athletes owing to biomechanical and hormonal inputs. Health providers need to be familiar with evidence-based evaluation, management, and emerging prevention strategies of these injuries.
- Exercising women, especially endurance athletes, are at heightened risk of depleting iron stores that can negatively impact athletic performance. Both iron deficiency nonanemia and iron deficiency anemia can be detected through history, examination, and lab indices, and can be effectively treated with early nutritional guidance.

INTRODUCTION

As decades have passed, and particularly with the passing of Title IX legislation, women are increasingly participating in more and more sporting activities. For years, women athletes have been treated as the "female" equivalent of male athletes, with

[a] Primary Care Sports Medicine Fellowship, Department of Family Medicine, University of Virginia Sports Medicine, University of Virginia Health System, Charlottesville, VA 22908-0729, USA; [b] Primary Care Sports Medicine Fellowship, Department of Physical Medicine & Rehabilitation, University of Virginia Sports Medicine, University of Virginia Health System, Charlottesville, VA 22908-0729, USA; [c] Department of Family Medicine, University of Virginia Health System, Charlottesville, VA 22908-0729, USA; [d] Department of Family Medicine, Faculty Development Fellowship, University of Virginia Health System, Charlottesville, VA 22908-0729, USA
* Corresponding author. Primary Care Sports Medicine Fellowship, Department of Family Medicine, University of Virginia Sports Medicine, University of Virginia Health System, Charlottesville, VA 22908-0729.
E-mail address: siobhan@virginia.edu

Prim Care Clin Office Pract 47 (2020) 65–85
https://doi.org/10.1016/j.pop.2019.11.002
0095-4543/20/© 2019 Elsevier Inc. All rights reserved.

similar medical approaches, but this is changing. The concept that women are unique in their "athletic arena" is further underscored with emerging scientific evidence from the physiologic details not visible to the eye, to the more overt biomechanical and anatomic differences. In this article, we review a handful of conditions that active women potentially may encounter: pregnancy, the female athlete triad, patellofemoral pain (PFP), potential injuries to the anterior cruciate ligament, and anemia.

EXERCISE AND PREGNANCY

The advantages of regular exercise to one's health are well established in the literature. Global recommendations, such as 150 minutes of moderate intensity exercise scattered over the course of a week, is considered standard when counseling patients. But what is the case for a pregnant woman? Both the US Department of Health and Human Services as well as the American College of Obstetrics and Gynecology (ACOG) encourage exercise in healthy pregnant women following consultation with a care provider. We will review the potential benefits and risks, as well as recommendations on how to approach exercise prescription.

Benefits

A woman's ability to exercise during pregnancy is affected by significant hormonal, metabolic, cardiovascular, pulmonary, musculoskeletal, thermoregulatory, and anatomic changes.[1,2] Maternal blood volume increases, as does heart rate and cardiac output, whereas systemic vascular resistance decreases. Oxygen consumption of the body climbs, yet pulmonary functional residual capacity and oxygen reserve decrease, resulting in increased minute ventilation. With physiologic changes such as these, initiating an exercise regimen or even continuing one may prove challenging. A stepwise approach is recommended; starting out slow and easy, ensuring excellent nutrition, rest and hydration, and later increasing exercise accordingly.

The benefits of exercise during pregnancy are widespread:[1]

- *Improved and/or maintained fitness*: pregnant women who exercised at least 2 to 3 times a week seemed to improve or maintain their level of fitness.[3] These benefits have been noted for cardiorespiratory and musculoskeletal endurance, aerobic fitness, and body composition.
- *Healthy weight gain*: the days of carte-blanche food consumption during pregnancy are long behind us, with different governing bodies making specific recommendations on what constitutes healthy gestational weight gain. These are based on prepregnancy weights and body mass indexes. Underweight women are encouraged to gain up to 40 pounds, whereas morbidly obese women are urged to limit weight gain to minimal amounts, if any. Instituting a regular exercise regimen will help moderate weight gain.[4]
- *Reduced gestational hypertension*: although the quality and strength of evidence is variable, exercising women may be less likely to develop hypertensive disorders during pregnancy than nonexercising subjects. There is no clear indication, however, that exercise prevents the development of preeclampsia across these same cohorts.[1]
- *Shortened labor*: recent studies suggest a reduced first stage labor for regular exercisers.[1]
- *Less risk of cesarean section*: exercising pregnant women are less likely to require cesarean section.[1]

- *Reduced musculoskeletal and pelvic floor pain*: routine weight-bearing exercise offers a protective effect relative to pregnancy changes that predispose women to back and/or pelvic floor pain.

Risks

Every individual has a unique personal medical history, and although exercise is beneficial during pregnancy, it may also pose certain risks. As a result, each patient must be well informed before initiation or continuation of specific activities (**Box 1**). Potential risks include trauma sustained to the mother, hyperthermia (particularly if exercise is completed in "hot environments," such as "hot yoga"), and reduced uteroplacental perfusion due to shunting to working muscle groups. Furthermore, because of physiologic changes during pregnancy, there is an increased risk of hypotension, particularly with supine positioning. Altered musculotendinous and joint laxity compounded by a shift in center of gravity can also predispose pregnant women to injury. Because many of these "pregnancy-induced alterations" occur in a subtle fashion, it is essential to ensure that the patient is aware of warning signs that warrant immediate discontinuation of exercise and urgent assessment by a care provider (**Box 2**). Educational handouts for patients are especially helpful as a written reference and reminder.

Box 1
Safe and unsafe physical activities during pregnancy

The following activities are safe to initiate or continue[a]:
- Walking
- Swimming
- Stationary cycling
- Low-impact aerobics
- Yoga, modified[b]
- Pilates, modified
- Running or jogging[c]
- Racquet sports[c,d]
- Strength training[c]

The following activities should be avoided:
- Contact sports (eg, ice hockey, boxing, soccer, and basketball)
- Activities with a high risk of falling (eg, downhill snow skiing, water skiing, surfing, off-road cycling, gymnastics, and horseback riding)
- Scuba diving
- Sky diving
- "Hot yoga" or "hot pilates"

[a] In women with uncomplicated pregnancies in consultation with an obstetric care provider.
[b] Yoga positions that result in decreased venous return and hypotension should be avoided as much as possible.
[c] In consultation with an obstetric care provider, running or jogging, racquet sports, and strength training may be safe for pregnant women who participated in these activities regularly before pregnancy.
[d] Racquet sports wherein a pregnant woman's changing balance may affect rapid movements and increase the risk of falling should be avoided as much as possible.
Reprinted with permission from Physical activity and exercise during pregnancy and the postpartum period. Committee Opinion No. 650. American College of Obstetricians and Gynecologists. Obstet Gynecol 2015:126:e135–42.

Box 2
Warning signs to discontinue exercise when pregnant

- Vaginal bleeding
- Regular painful contractions
- Amniotic fluid leakage
- Dyspnea before exertion
- Dizziness
- Headache
- Chest pain
- Muscle weakness affecting balance
- Calf pain or swelling

Reprinted with permission from Physical activity and exercise during pregnancy and the postpartum period. Committee Opinion No. 650. American College of Obstetricians and Gynecologists. Obstet Gynecol 2015:126:e135–42.

Exercise Prescription

Women who participate in regular exercise frequently hope to continue activity into pregnancy. Interestingly, nonexercisers frequently become more receptive to healthier lifestyle choices as they realize they are potentially affecting the health of their offspring. Therefore, care providers should be prepared to take advantage of this opportunity by having the necessary knowledge to safely advise and encourage pregnant patients about exercise regimens.

Before the approval of exercise continuation or initiation, it is imperative to determine maternal and fetal risk. This assessment includes a thorough review of medical history, ongoing health concerns, current and previous pregnancy-related complications, medications, family history, an assessment of current physical activity level, followed by a detailed clinical examination. The American College of Sports Medicine's Health-Related Physical Fitness Assessment is a helpful resource to guide this screening and prescription process.[5] Absolute and relative contraindications must be ruled out (**Boxes 3** and **4**) and patients should be provided with a list of safe exercises, as well as those to avoid. Education regarding parameters on exercise intensity, progression, frequency, duration, and warm up and cool down are necessary to review. In the past, maternal pulse rates were used as a metric for patient exertion. However, ACOG now recommends that patients use their *perceived exertion* rating as a self-guide.[6] Level of exertion can be quantified to a score of 13 to 14 on the Borg Rating of Perceived Exertion scale. Alternatively, a simple "talk test" serves similar function: if able to carry on a normal conversation, the intensity is deemed low to moderate. On the other hand, if speaking becomes difficult, the exertion level is likely too high. Proper hydration leading up to, during, and following exercise is also a key point to address, as this can have significant effects on both maternal and fetal circulation. Again, starting out slow with lower intensity exercises is most prudent to allow for a gentle adaptation to increased physical exertion.

In the postpartum period, exercise should be encouraged as soon as it is safe, as benefits can be both physical and mental. When coupled with a healthy postpartum diet, exercise can promote weight loss and help to prevent the development of obesity and comorbid metabolic disorders. As long as the exercise is enjoyable, physical

---

Box 3
Absolute contraindications to aerobic exercise during pregnancy

- Hemodynamically significant heart disease
- Restrictive lung disease
- Incompetent cervix or cerclage
- Multiple gestation at risk of premature labor
- Persistent second- or third-trimester bleeding
- Placenta previa after 26 weeks of gestation
- Premature labor during the current pregnancy
- Ruptured membranes
- Preeclampsia or pregnancy-induced hypertension
- Severe anemia

Reprinted with permission from Physical activity and exercise during pregnancy and the postpartum period. Committee Opinion No. 650. American College of Obstetricians and Gynecologists. Obstet Gynecol 2015;126:e135–42.

---

activity has been associated with a decreased risk of postpartum depression, although further studies in this area are needed.

FEMALE ATHLETE TRIAD
Definition

The female athlete triad (FAT) is a condition in physically active women manifested by the interrelationship of 3 elements: (1) low energy availability (intake minus

---

Box 4
Relative contraindications to aerobic exercise during pregnancy

- Anemia
- Unevaluated maternal cardiac arrhythmia
- Chronic bronchitis
- Poorly controlled type 1 diabetes
- Extreme morbid obesity
- Extreme underweight (BMI <12)
- History of extremely sedentary lifestyle
- Intrauterine growth restriction in current pregnancy
- Poorly controlled hypertension
- Orthopedic limitations
- Poorly controlled seizure disorder
- Poorly controlled hyperthyroidism
- Heavy smoker

Reprinted with permission from Physical activity and exercise during pregnancy and the postpartum period. Committee Opinion No. 650. American College of Obstetricians and Gynecologists. Obstet Gynecol 2015;126:e135–42.

expenditure) with or without disordered eating, (2) menstrual dysfunction, and (3) low bone mineral density (BMD). Disordered eating includes a spectrum of behaviors: restrictive eating; fasting; frequently skipped meals; use of diet pills, laxatives, diuretics, and/or enemas; overeating; bingeing and purging; and clinically defined eating disorders. Menstrual dysfunction may include oligomenorrhea (cycles >35 days); luteal suppression (luteal phase <11 days or with low concentration of progesterone); anovulation (cycle without ovulation); or amenorrhea (no menstrual cycle for >90 days). Low BMD is defined as a BMD Z score between −1.0 and −2.0.[7]

FAT is typically considered along a spectrum, and affected individuals may not reflect symptoms in all 3 areas simultaneously. However, this condition can lead to longstanding negative health outcomes. Therefore, it is important to consider when addressing the health of female athletes, particularly if there are opportunities to intervene early.[8] Primary care clinicians are often on the front lines of its assessment, yet a study from 2015 demonstrated that only 47% of medicine, pediatric, and family physicians had knowledge of the triad.[9]

Within the past 5 years, a new term has been proposed that expands the female triad to include a broader syndrome affecting men also—Relative Energy Deficiency in Sport (RED-S). Although the International Olympic Committee has issued several position statements on RED-S, the true nature of RED-S is still under some debate and ongoing study.

Prevalence

The reported prevalence of FAT is highly variable (range from 0% to 54%)[10] and often challenging to address, as certain elements may be considered the "norm" for the sport. For example, evidence is strong that disordered eating and menstrual dysfunction may be especially prevalent among women who participate in sports that emphasize "leanness," for example, lightweight rowing, gymnastics, dance, figure skating, cheerleading, distance running, and pole vaulting.

Risk Factors

Multiple risk factors are associated with the various components of FAT and are well outlined in various evidence-based reviews.[10,11] Risk factors include sport type, psychosocial issues, dietary and nutritional issues, body image, training regimen, and health history, to name a few.

Diagnosis

Because of the highly interrelated nature of the triad, it is important for primary care clinicians to understand how the various components relate to each other, with particular focus on where the various components for an individual are occurring along the spectrum of optimal health to pathology. In addition, although there is a greater risk association for certain sports, various components of the triad may be present for individuals participating in any sport and should be considered during opportunities for contact with a health care provider during preparticipation physicals and annual examinations.

Although there is not strong evidence regarding the benefits of screening questions, the Triad Consensus Panel recommends asking screening questions during preparticipation physicals. These questions are also relevant during other health examinations also. Further examination is warranted if the individual seems to possess any one of the triad components:[8]

Triad Screening Questions

- Have you ever had a menstrual period?
- How old were you when you had your first menstrual period?
- When was your most recent menstrual period?
- How many periods have you had in the past 12 months?
- Are you presently taking any female hormones (estrogen, progesterone, birth control pills)?
- Do you worry about your weight?
- Are you trying to or has anyone recommended that you gain or lose weight?
- Are you on a special diet or do you avoid certain types of foods or food groups?
- Have you ever had an eating disorder?
- Have you ever had a stress fracture?
- Have you ever been told you have low bone density (osteopenia or osteoporosis)?

The physical examination should address associated risk factors, including the patient's body mass index (BMI), weight history, presence of orthostatic hypotension, as well as other physical manifestations of eating disorders, for example, presence of lanugo, parotid gland swelling, and calluses on the proximal interphalangeal joints.[8] The BMI of pediatric patients should be interpreted carefully and adjusted according to age and gender estimates until the age of 20 years. In addition, body weight should not be the only marker used to assess energy availability.[8] If energy deficiency is suspected, assessment by a nutritionist (particularly a sports dietician) is warranted as there are accuracy issues in both the reporting and interpretation of food logs.[8] If an eating disorder is suspected, it is helpful to include a mental health professional in the care of the patient. When primary or secondary amenorrhea is present, it is important to rule out pregnancy or possible endocrinopathies. Regarding suspected low BMD, a dual-energy X-ray absorptiometry scan may be indicated based on the patient's risk stratification (moderate to high risk) and presence of previous stress fractures. A full explanation of the risk stratification can be found in the 2014 Female Athlete Triad Coalition Consensus Statement.[8]

Treatment

Preliminary treatment efforts typically focus on nonpharmacologic approaches. Primary goals of the treatment plan are to increase the patient's energy availability, restore her body weight, and restore menses.[12] However, the Consensus Panel highlighted the importance of incorporating the goals of the patient, her training regimen, dietary needs, and other relevant contextual variables.[8] One of the first places to begin treatment is to address the patient's energy availability by enhancing her nutritional status and decreasing her energy expenditure by modifying her exercise behavior. Depending on the severity, this could include reducing the training regimen and a reduction or restriction from competition. In addition, the psychosocial component of the treatment process must be considered. For example, among highly competitive gymnasts, physical manifestations of sexual maturity may be viewed negatively.[13] For a treatment regimen to succeed, it is important to address the patient's thoughts around body image, attitudes toward food intake, as well as knowledge around energy needs associated with a given sport. Depending on the nature of the patient's condition and age, a broader team approach is often needed, including a dietician/sports nutritionist, exercise physiologist, mental health provider, and her parents and/or coach.[10]

There are no universally accepted guidelines related to FAT regarding clearance and when patients may return to their sport.[8] Utilizing the Consensus Panel risk stratification may be somewhat useful, particularly as it relates to bone health and potential for fracture, but it is important to interpret the results according to the individual patient and her context.

PATELLOFEMORAL PAIN
Definition

PFP is a common condition. Patients may present with peripatellar pain and/or retropatellar pain. Secondary, but "nonessential" presentations may include crepitus or a grinding sensation within the knee during flexion; tenderness when palpating the patellar facets; a small effusion; and/or pain when seated or when rising after being seated.[14] Typically, pain is not experienced when the patellofemoral joint is not loaded.[15] This condition can have long-standing effects on an individual's ability to participate in pain-free physical activity, as 50% or more of those individuals with a diagnosis of PFP may continue to experience symptoms 5 years or more after their diagnosis.[16]

Prevalence

The annual prevalence is approximately 23% in adults and 29% in adolescents. The estimated point prevalence in female athletes is approximately 23%,[17] and a 10% incidence rate has been reported in reference to middle- and high-school female basketball players.[18] Of particular note, 1 study demonstrated that women were 2.23 times more likely to develop PFP than men.[19]

Cause

Biomechanical factors
Biomechanical explanations relate to forces that are exerted on the patella that affect its tracking within the trochlear groove. These forces occur due to pelvic instability, internal rotation of the femur, valgus forces on the knee, internal rotation of the tibia, and/or foot protonation. Reduced strength of the quadriceps muscles and diminished activation of the vastus medialis oblique have been discussed in the literature as possible culprits, although there may be differences across adult versus adolescent populations. Specifically, adults with PFP may have a weakness in their quadriceps, whereas this association has not been demonstrated among adolescents.[20] This finding has potential implications when considering exercise therapy as a treatment modality for adolescent patients.[16] However, if an adolescent with PFP possesses quadriceps strength deficits, strength training may still be appropriate.

As with quadriceps strength, there is also debate regarding the association of hip strength with PFP,[20] although hip biomechanics may be more relevant to PFP among women than men.[21] A recent study found that 52% of women with PFP were likely to present with 2 or more kinematic alterations: peak hip adduction, peak knee flexion, and peak rearfoot eversion. Furthermore, a positive association was found between the number of kinematic alterations and a higher pain level, as well as a negative association between the number of kinematic alterations and functional status.[22]

Structural causes
The Q-angle is the vector formed by 2 lines; the line from the center of the patella to the anterior superior iliac spine, and an extended line from the center of the patella through the tibial tubercle (**Fig. 1**). The Q-angle is related to patellar tracking and has been considered in relation to PFP. However, patellar tracking is also affected by the location of an individual's anatomic structures, various forces acting on those structures,

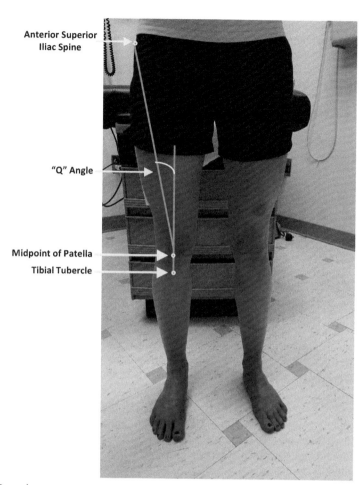

Fig. 1. Q-angle.

as well as the relative strength of the different quadriceps muscles. Current data suggest that the Q-angle alone does not appear to be associated with the development of PFP.[23]

Static alignment

Data surrounding the impact of static alignment of the rearfoot, foot protonation, and pelvic drop on PFP remains conflicting and warrants minimal consideration when assessing patients with PFP.[16] Overall, the relationship between structural deficits and PFP is inconsistent. Although the assessment of underlying structures, especially through imaging, may be indicated for certain patients, the impact of imaging on treatment decisions for PFP is limited.[16]

Diagnosis

PFP can arise from multiple factors, although joint loading activities tend to exacerbate PFP. These include squats, climbing or descending stairs, and sports that involve running, cycling, and sitting for prolonged periods of time.[24] It is important to take a multidimensional approach to the assessment process, which includes an assessment of the patient's biomechanics, gaining an understanding of the patient's history of joint load and intensity of physical activity, as well as understanding the patient's attitudes toward physical activity and the associated discomfort.[16]

Much of the diagnostic challenge of PFP is due to the multiple etiologic factors of this condition and a corresponding lack of definitive diagnostic criteria. A systematic review of clinical PFP diagnostic tests revealed variable outcomes due to inconsistent approaches (**Table 1**).[25] The *patellar tilt test* and the *squat test* showed the best "trend" toward diagnosing PFP and, overall, the squat test was deemed one of the better diagnostic tests, although still not a definitive test. The *vastus medialis coordination test* was among the highest specificity tests (93% specific) but the sensitivity was low (16% sensitivity). Medial and lateral facet tenderness on palpation was also present in 71% to 74% of those with PFP. There was limited evidence that combining multiple diagnostic tests was superior to any individual test.

Gathering subjective information is necessary, with particular focus on gaining an understanding of the nature of the patient's physical activity, frequency, and intensity. Is the patient involved with organized sports? If yes, for how long? How frequently is the patient exercising and at what duration and intensity? How might the patient's activities be influenced by the patient's aspirations, coaches, and parents, when relevant? What is the training regimen and does it allow for sufficient recovery? All of this must be considered when assessing the patient and developing a management plan.[16]

Other conditions should also be considered in the evaluation of anterior knee pain. For example, Epocrates provides a useful table within their differential diagnosis section for Patellofemoral Pain Syndrome that includes a variety of diseases/conditions, along with associated signs, symptoms and related testing).[15,26]

Management

Recommendations for PFP management based on the evidence and expert panels have remained relatively consistent within recent years.[24,27] Low quality but consistent evidence for exercise therapy in addressing pain and improving function is present.[28] However, there is insufficient evidence to guide providers regarding which specific exercises to prescribe. Based on the 2018 Consensus Statement from the Patellofemoral Pain Research Retreat, recommendations were made for PFP management (**Table 2**):[24]

Exercise prescriptions may include open kinetic chain (OKC) activities (eg, leg curls) and closed kinetic chain (CKC) activities (eg, leg press). Expert providers prefer CKC

Table 1						
Test characteristics of patellofemoral examination maneuvers						
Test	**Sensitivity %**	**Specificity %**	**+ Likelihood Ratio**	**– Likelihood Ratio**	**+ Predictive Value**	**– Predictive Value**
Patellar tilt	43	92	5.4	0.6	93	40
Squats	91	50	1.8	0.2	79	74
Vastus medialis coordination	16	93	2.3	0.9	71	50
Medial tenderness	48	71	1.6	0.7	74	44
Lateral tenderness	41	71	1.4	0.8	71	41

Data from Nunes GS, Stapait EL, Kirsten MH, et al. Clinical test for diagnosis of patellofemoral pain syndrome: systematic review with meta-analysis. Phys Ther in Sport 2013;14:54-9.

Table 2
2018 Consensus statement from the patellofemoral pain research retreat recommendations for patellofemoral pain management

Approach	Short Term	Medium Term	Long Term
Exercise Therapy			
Pain reduction	X	X	X
Improved function and symptoms	Uncertain	X	X
Combined Hip and Knee Therapy			
Pain reduction	X	X	X
Improved function and symptoms	X	X	X
Hip Targeted Therapy (compared with knee targeted)			
Pain reduction	Uncertain	Uncertain	Uncertain
Improved function and symptoms	Uncertain	Uncertain	Uncertain
Combined Interventions			
Pain reduction	X	X	Uncertain among adolescents
Improved function and symptoms			
Prefabricated Foot Orthoses			
Pain reduction	X		
Improved function	Uncertain		
Patellar Taping			
Pain reduction	Uncertain when taping only		Uncertain when combining taping with exercise
Bracing			
Pain reduction	Uncertain	Uncertain	

Adapted from Collins NJ, Barton CJ, van Middelkoop M, et al. 2018 consensus statement on exercise therapy and physical interventions (orthoses, taping and manual therapy) to treat patellofemoral pain: recommendations from the 5th International Patellofemoral Pain Research Retreat, Gold Coast, Australia, 2017. Br J Sports Med. 2018;52:1174; with permission.

activities, although they highlight OKC activities during the early stages of rehabilitation, as these more effectively target specific muscle groups (eg, vastus medialis oblique).[29] Although much of the exercise therapy focus is on addressing strength deficits in the quadriceps and hips, building true muscle strength beyond the improved neural changes takes time (minimum of 6 weeks). Low to moderate resistance training may be useful and ultimately, although it can be started at home, may be best addressed through a gym-based program focusing on progressing activity for a minimum of 2 times per week over at least a 6-month period.[16] The use of prefabricated foot orthoses may also reduce short-term pain. At present, there is no evidence that custom orthotics are superior and it is not clear which patients may benefit most given their foot structure and function.[24]

A variety of adjunctive interventions are available, but data to support these treatment approaches are either uncertain or deemed inappropriate (**Table 3**):[24]

Table 3
Adjunctive interventions for patellofemoral pain

Approach	Recommendation
Acupuncture or dry needling to trigger points	Uncertain
Patellofemoral and knee mobilization	Inappropriate
Lumbar mobilization/manipulation	Inappropriate
Electrophysical agents (eg, ultrasound, phonophoresis, and laser therapy)	Inappropriate
Manual soft tissue techniques (eg, ischemic compression to peripatellar and retropatellar trigger points; myofascial techniques)	Uncertain
Blood flow restriction training	Uncertain
Gait retraining	Uncertain

Adapted from Collins NJ, Barton CJ, van Middelkoop M, et al. 2018 consensus statement on exercise therapy and physical interventions (orthoses, taping and manual therapy) to treat patellofemoral pain: recommendations from the 5th International Patellofemoral Pain Research Retreat, Gold Coast, Australia, 2017. Br J Sports Med. 2018;52:1174; with permission.

Although evidence is lacking regarding a definitive diagnostic and treatment approach to PFP, providers do have options. Given the multifactorial nature of PFP, a patient-centered approach tailored to individual needs is warranted. In addition, given the likely chronicity of this condition and often lengthy rehabilitation process, it is important to actively address patient expectations and to use shared decision making when developing a treatment plan.[16]

ANTERIOR CRUCIATE LIGAMENT INJURIES IN THE FEMALE ATHLETE
Epidemiology/Risk Factors

Noncontact anterior cruciate ligament (ACL) injuries occur 2 to 10 times more frequently in female athletes compared with men across all skill levels.[30–32] In female athletes, rates of noncontact ACL injury increase after the onset of puberty, occurring in the late teenage years to early 20s while participating in sports requiring abrupt shifts in momentum (eg, basketball, soccer). This is distinct from contact ACL injuries, which occur at similar rates across genders. The increased noncontact ACL injury rate is thought to be multifactorial:[30,31,33]

- Hormonal: estrogen-induced ligamentous laxity and changes in neuromuscular control with highest rate of ACL tears during preovulatory days 9 to 14.
- Anatomic: increased Q-angle, narrow intercondylar arch.
- Biomechanical: imbalanced quad-to-hamstring strength ratio, gluteal weakness, landing position with more upright posturing than men, physiologic rotational laxity of lower extremity.
- Environmental: footwear and surface.

Long-term, ACL injuries commonly predispose an individual, regardless of sex, to debilitating knee sequelae such as instability, meniscal injuries, and knee osteoarthritis.[30,31,33]

Mechanism of Injury/Clinical Manifestation

ACL injuries occur most often during abrupt stops, landing, or cutting with *VROOM* positioning: *V*algus positioning of knee, externally *R*otated leg, flat f*O*oted, and *O*ut of control *M*ovement (**Fig. 2**). Following such a mechanical load, the athlete may report the sensation of a "pop," knee instability, "giving way," or quick-onset knee pain and swelling. These symptoms should increase suspicion for an acute ACL injury and trigger further investigation.[30–33]

Evaluation

Evaluation begins with a targeted history including pointed inquiry into any features that increase likelihood of an ACL injury: audible or subjective knee pop, instability, rapid effusion, or pain. There exists a time-sensitive nature to performing the physical examination with greater accuracy to avoid the onset of increased swelling, pain, and subsequent guarding and protective muscle action. The examination must note any degree of effusion, active and passive range of motion, areas of focal tenderness, palpable defects, neurovascular status, and special tests. Special tests such as the Lachman maneuver, anterior drawer sign, Lelli lever sign test, and/or Pivot-shift (**Table 4**) significantly aid the examiner in accurately detecting ACL injuries. Of these, the Lachman maneuver and Pivot-shift test have shown superior test performance.[34] When the Lachman maneuver provides equivocal results, the addition of other special tests may add further clinical value.

If further evaluation is required after examination, MR imaging is the gold standard yielding an 87% sensitivity and 91% specificity for detection of ACL injuries. A

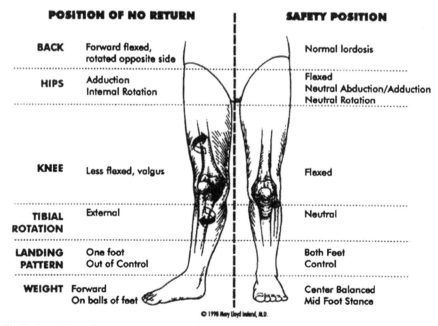

Fig. 2. Depiction of components of VROOM posturing: ACL injuries occur most often during abrupt stops, landing, or cutting with *VROOM* positioning: *V*algus positioning of knee, externally *R*otated leg, flat f*O*oted, and *O*ut of control *M*ovement. (Ireland ML. Anterior cruciate ligament injury in female athletes: epidemiology. J Athl Train. 1999;34(2):152; with permission.)

| Table 4 | | |
| Likelihood ratios of anterior cruciate ligament special tests on examination | | |
ACL Special Test	Positive Likelihood Ratio	Negative Likelihood Ratio
Lachman maneuver	12	0.14
Pivot-shift test	20	0.4
Lelli lever sign test	6.3	0.41
Anterior drawer sign	3.7	0.6

preliminary knee radiograph may be considered in the setting of an acute knee injury, but clinical criteria are available to aid primary care providers in knowing when *not* to order radiographs. The Ottawa knee rules (sensitivity 100%, specificity 52%) allow providers to forego knee radiographs when a patient suffers an acute knee injury as long as none of the following criteria are met:

- Age >55 years
- Fibular head tenderness
- Isolated patellar tenderness
- Inability to flex >90°
- Inability to walk >4 steps[34]

Management

Prompt initiation of physical therapy targeted to relieve pain, swelling, and loss of stability/function are crucial once the diagnosis of an ACL injury has been made. Conservative therapies should be initiated regardless of planned surgery and include nonsteroidal anti-inflammatory drugs (NSAIDs), ice, elevation, rest, bracing, and physical therapy. Factors, such as the degree of ACL tearing (partial versus complete), patient age, desired postinjury activity, preinjury level of sport, and any coexisting injuries, determines the need early surgical consultation or intervention.[34,35] However, recent controlled trials have discovered that structured rehabilitation with conservative therapies assists 2 of 3 young, active adults presenting with isolated, acute ACL injuries in a previously healthy knee avoid reconstructive surgery with no differences in functional outcomes or quality of life.[36]

Prevention

For decades, research has sought to identify modifiable risk factors for ACL injuries in female athletes. Current literature highlights the primary targets of ACL injury prevention as landing techniques and neuromuscular recruitment. Low to moderate quality evidence suggests multimodal prevention programs composed of muscle strengthening and recruitment, landing drills, proprioception, and plyometrics may significantly reduce rates of noncontact ACL injuries.[37] Such a program would ideally be implemented at or before puberty, start 6 weeks preseason, occur 2 to 3 times weekly, continue throughout the season in place of 15- to 20-minute warm ups, and provide feedback of mechanics. Primary muscles of interest for strengthening include hip abductors (eg, gluteus maximus and medius), hamstrings, and core muscles that are able to counteract VROOM positioning.

The most well-studied and popular prevention programs over the past 2 decades have a calculated number needed to treat of 70 to 100 to prevent 1 noncontact ACL injury in women.[37] This gives the primary care provider more understanding of how wide-scale, population-based implementation of such programs can potentially reduce the burden of disease in young, active women. In addition, preliminary data suggest that these ACL prevention programs improve athletic performance by enhancing single leg hop distance, vertical jump, sprint speed, and squat strength; such improvements in athletic performance may increase compliance with a prevention program by players and coaches alike. Future studies are needed to clarify which components of these prevention programs are most effective at decreasing injury rates and improving athletic performance.[37,38]

IRON/ANEMIA IN THE FEMALE ATHLETE
Epidemiology/Risk Factors

Iron is an essential micronutrient for life, especially for the exercising athlete. The body requires iron in increasing quantities during periods of rapid growth, training recovery, high altitude training, menstruation, foot-strike hemolysis secondary to running, and injury recovery.[39] It is estimated that 24% to 47% of exercising women have iron deficiency without anemia, otherwise called iron deficiency non-anemia (IDNA) and occurs approximately twice as frequently in exercising women compared with the general population. Current evidence reveals that both iron-deficient anemia (IDA) and IDNA inhibit muscle work capacity, immune function, metabolic efficiency, cognitive function, tissue training adaptation, and athletic performance.[40] Particular athletes at increased risk of iron deficiency are female athletes (having iron needs that may be >70% of average dietary requirements), endurance athletes (eg, distance runners), vegetarians, and athletes with eating disorders.[39]

Physiology, Pathophysiology, and Clinical Manifestations

Iron is most readily absorbed from heme-containing compounds in the small intestine. In the duodenum, iron is processed by enterocytes, carried across the cellular membrane by ferroportin (a hepcidin-inhibited transport protein), and delivered throughout the body via transferrin (**Fig. 3**). Estrogen inhibits hepcidin activity thereby increasing enteral absorption of bioavailable iron.[40]

Importantly, iron is also absorbed in proportion to the number of calories in one's diet; research has demonstrated that 6 mg of iron is absorbed per 1000 kcal. Therefore, suboptimal ingestion of total calories or heme-containing food sources can lead to negative iron balances.[39] This may occur through intentional dietary restriction or via a phenomenon termed "inadvertent undereating." More common in women than men, inadvertent undereating is a state in which postexercise energy deficiency leads to decreased appetite by suppressing low orexigenic molecules (eg, ghrelin) and leads to increased satiety.[40] Regardless of the cause, negative iron balance can manifest in a myriad of ways (**Box 5**).[41]

An additional cause of the anemic state in a training athlete is "sports anemia"—a transient, aerobic training-induced hemodilution that decreases hemoglobin levels but corrects without intervention as sport continues. Rather than a pathologic phenomenon, sports anemia actually seems to hold beneficial value in adapting to aerobic training. However, any persistent anemia should be considered pathologic and corrected promptly.[39]

Evaluation/Treatment

Based on current evidence, it is recommended to reserve IDA screening for at-risk populations (eg, female athletes, distance runners, vegetarians, athletes practicing

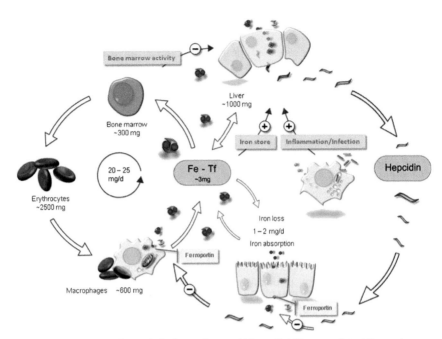

Fig. 3. The regulation of iron (Fe) absorption and bioavailability: regulated through a negative feedback loop that centers on the ferroportin-inhibiting activity of hepcidin, a protein produced in the liver in response to increasing iron stores or inflammation due to infection or other stressors (ie, exercise). This highlights how increasing exercise loads may inhibit iron absorption via inflammation and increased hepcidin production. (*From* Kemna EHJM. Hepcidine regulatie. Available at: https://commons.wikimedia.org/wiki/File:Hepcidine_regulatie.jpg.)

vegan diets, and athletes with eating disorders). This is in contrast to limiting diagnostic evaluation of anemia for symptomatic athletes (see symptom list above). Lab studies to detect IDA include complete blood count, serum ferritin, and iron indices (includes serum iron, transferrin, and percent transferrin saturation).

Screening/evaluation key points

- Normative values of ferritin tend to be low, for example, less than 5 ng/mL. Consensus for normal ferritin levels in active, exercising women is ≥ 15 to 35 ng/mL; notably, a more precise consensus exists for normal hemoglobin levels and is ≥ 12 g/dL.[42,43]
- Noniron-deficient causes of fatigue should be evaluated and optimized. These include underlying illness, inflammatory conditions, poor sleep, negative work-to-recovery balance, and education/work/family/social-related stressors.

Management

IDNA (low ferritin, normal hemoglobin): treatment begins with dietary education and referral to a sports dietician. The female athlete should aim to consume both an iron-rich (containing >18 mg of elemental iron per day) and vitamin C-rich diet. Athletes

---

Box 5
Signs of low iron availability

- Decreased athletic performance
- Fatigue
- Palpitations
- Dyspnea
- Glossitis
- Angular stomatitis
- Pica
- Koilonychia
- Blue sclera
- Esophageal webbing (Plummer-Vinson syndrome)
- Bone stress injuries
- Recurrent sport-related injuries
- Prolonged injury recovery
- Impaired growth/adaptation
- Menstrual irregularities
- Decreased fertility
- Poor concentration
- Decreased maximal oxygen uptake (Vo_2 max)

---

should be advised to decrease wheat intake, calcium and phosphorus supplements, antacids, and NSAIDs at the time of iron-containing meals because these potentially inhibit enteral uptake of iron. In addition to dietary adjustments, it can be beneficial to evaluate and address training loads. If a high training load is present, consider reducing the regimen; examples of load reduction may include rest from vigorous or endurance exercise or descent from high altitude. Some additional key points include:

- The most readily absorbable sources of iron include eggs (especially egg yolks), liver, lean red meat (especially beef), oysters, poultry, salmon, tuna, and shellfish. Lesser but appreciable amounts are absorbed from dried beans (lima, soy, kidney), dried fruits (prunes, raisins, apricots), iron-fortified cereals, green vegetables (broccoli, spinach, kale, asparagus), almonds, and whole grains.
- Iron indices may take 3 to 6 months to restore with diet alone.
- Repeat hematologic indices in 1 to 3 months after initiating interventions.[42]
- A trial of oral iron supplementation can be considered in IDNA to normalize iron status (eg, ferritin levels). There exist conflicting data that supplementation may improve athletic performance and training load tolerance in female IDNA endurance athletes.[42] However, several randomized clinical trials have shown no improvement in performance with oral or intravenous iron supplementation versus placebo in female IDNA endurance athletes when serum ferritin reaches levels as low as 30 μg/L.[42]
- Iron supplementation should be taken apart from meals and in combination with oral vitamin C 500 mg once daily.

- Supplementation should occur only under medical supervision to monitor risks and benefits. A common side effect is that of significant gastrointestinal (GI) distress such as constipation, cramping, or bloating. To minimize these, consider low-dose ferrous sulfate (125 mg) or minimize the frequency of intake (eg, once daily, biweekly).
- Response to iron therapy should be monitored with serum iron indices once every 2 to 4 weeks. Results should be documented and guide further therapy.[42]
- *Caveat*: there is no agreement on a single ferritin value to identify a problematic iron deficiency state. Clinical judgment is necessary as ferritin is considered an acute phase reactant. If an inflammatory state is suspected in an athlete, ferritin values may appear within normal ranges instead of revealing the true iron deficiency.

IDA (low hemoglobin): Before initiating therapy, the medical provider should verify that a full history, review of systems, and physical examination has been completed to identify and correct any secondary causes of anemia (eg, abnormal menstrual bleeding, GI blood loss, or insufficient dietary iron intake). The approach to treating IDA is multifactorial and includes dietary, behavioral, and medicinal components. The athlete should be instructed to consume an iron-rich, vitamin C-rich diet. Simultaneously referring the athlete to a sports dietician and initiating oral iron repletion (eg, oral ferrous sulfate 325 mg once or twice daily) is essential. Ideally, oral iron therapy should be consumed at a time remote from meals to increase enteral absorption, but GI intolerance may occur. Again, strategies to mitigate these include taking oral iron therapy with food or decreasing the dose of therapy, recognizing that these changes may decrease enteral iron absorption. Response to iron therapy can be determined by completing iron indices every 2 to 4 weeks, recognizing that it can take 3 to 6 months to reverse iron deficiency anemia in active athletes. Taking iron supplements immediately after strenuous exercise should be discouraged as optimal iron acquisition can be antagonized by physiologic, postexercise increases in hepcidin. Thus, it may be prudent to consider reducing training load, especially in the setting of erythrocyte hemolysis.

DISCLOSURE

The authors have nothing to disclose.

REFERENCES

1. Gregg VH, Fergusson JE. Exercise in pregnancy. In: the female athlete. Clin Sports Med 2017;36(4):741–52.
2. Bo K, Artal R, Barakat R, et al. Exercise and pregnancy in recreational and elite athletes: 2016/2017 evidence summary from the IOC expert group meeting, Lausanne. Part 5. Recommendations for health professionals and active women. Br J Sports Med 2018;52(17):1080–5.
3. Kramer MS, McDonald SW. Aerobic exercise for women during pregnancy. Cochrane Database Syst Rev 2006;(3):CD000180.
4. Muktabhant B, Lawrie TZ, Lumbiganon P, et al. Diet or exercise, or both, for preventing excessive weight gain in pregnancy. Cochrane Database Syst Rev 2015;(6):CD007145.
5. American College of Sports Medicine. ACSM's health-related physical fitness assessment manual. 5th edition. Philadelphia: Wolters Kluwer; 2017.

6. ACOG Committee Opinion No. 650: physical activity and exercise during pregnancy and the postpartum period. Obstet Gynecol 2015;126(6):e135–42. Reaffirmed 2017.

7. Nativ A, Loucks AB, Manore MM, et al. American College of Sports Medicine. American College of Sports Medicine Position Stand: the female athlete triad. Med Sci Sports Exerc 2007;39(10):1867–82.

8. DeSouza MJ, Nattiv A, Joy E, et al. 2014 female athlete triad coalition consensus statement on treatment and return to play of the female athlete triad. Br J Sports Med 2014;48:289.

9. Curry EJ, Logan C, Ackerman K, et al. Female athlete triad awareness among multispecialty physicians. Sports Med 2015;1:38.

10. Female athlete triad—DynaMed plus. Available at: http://www.dynamed.com/topics/dmp~AN~T922488/Female-athlete-triad. Accessed June 28, 2018.

11. Female athletic triad syndrome—essential evidence plus. Available at: http://www.essentialevidenceplus.com/content/eee/237. Accessed February 15, 2019.

12. Chamberlain R. The female athlete triad: recommendations for management. Am Fam Physician 2018;97(8):501–2.

13. Tan JOA, Calitri R, Bloodworth A, et al. Understanding eating disorders in elite gymnastics: ethical and conceptual challenges. Clin Sports Med 2016;35:275–92.

14. Crossley KM, Stefanik JJ, Selfe J, et al. 2016 Patellofemoral pain consensus statement from the 4th International Patellofemoral Pain Research Retreat, Manchester. Part 1: terminology, definitions, clinical examination, natural history, patellofemoral osteoarthritis and patient-reported outcome measures. Br J Sports Med 2016;50:839–43.

15. Crossley KM, Callaghan MJ, van Linschoten R. Patellofemoral pain. BMJ 2015;351:h3939.

16. Lack S, Neal B, De Oliveira Silva D, et al. How to manage patellofemoral pain: understanding the multifactorial nature and treatment options. Phys Ther Sport 2018;32:155–66.

17. Smith BE, Selfe J, Thacker D, et al. Incidence and prevalence of patellofemoral pain: a systematic review and meta-analysis. PLoS One 2018;13(1):e0190892.

18. Myer GD, Ford KR, Barber Foss KD, et al. The incidence and potential pathomechanics of patellofemoral pain in female athletes. Clin Biomech 2010;25:700–7.

19. Boling M, Padua D, Marshall S, et al. Gender differences in the incidence and prevalence of patellofemoral pain syndrome. Scand J Med Sci Sports 2010;20(5):725–30.

20. Rathleff SR, Baird WN, Olesen JL, et al. Hip and knee strength is not affected in 12-16 year old adolescents with patellofemoral pain: a cross-sectional population based study. PLoS One 2013;8(11):e79153.

21. Willy RW, Manal KT, Witvrouw EE, et al. Are mechanics different between male and female runnders with patellofemoral pain? Med Sci Sports Exerc 2012. https://doi.org/10.1249/MSS.0b013e3182629215.

22. Ferrari D, Briani RV, de Oliveira Silva D, et al. Higher pain level and lower functional capacity are associated with the number of altered kinematics in women with patellofemoral pain. Gait Posture 2018;60:268–72.

23. Boling MC, Nguyen AD, Padua DA, et al. Gender-specific risk factor profiles for patellofemoral pain. Clin J Sport Med 2019;00:1–8.

24. Collins NJ, Barton CJ, vanMiddelkoop M, et al. 2018 Consensus statement on exercise therapy and physical interventions (orthoses, taping and manual therapy)

to treat patellofemoral pain: recommendations from the 5th International Patellofemoral Pain Research Retreat, Gold Coast, Australia, 2017. Br J Sports Med 2018; 52:1170–8.

25. Nunes GS, Stapait EL, Kirsten MH, et al. Clinical test for diagnosis of patellofemoral pain syndrome: systematic review with meta-analysis. Phys Ther Sport 2013;14:54–9.

26. Epocrates patellofemoral pain syndrome: differential diagnosis. Available at: https://online.epocrates.com/diseases/82735/Patellofemoral-pain-syndrome/Differential-Diagnosis. Accessed January 30, 19.

27. Crossley KM, van Middelkoop M, Callaghan MJ, et al. 2016 Patellofemoral pain consensus statement from the 4th International Patellofemoral Pain Research Retreat, Manchester. Part 2: recommended physical interventions (exercise, taping, bracing, foot orthoses and combined interventions). Br J Sports Med 2016; 50:844–52.

28. Van der Heijden RA, Lankhorst NE, van Linschoten R, et al. Exercise for treating patellofemoral pain syndrome. Cochrane Database Syst Rev 2015;(1): CD010387.

29. Barton CJ, Lack S, Hemmings S, et al. The 'Best practice guide to conservative management of patellofemoral pain': incorporating level 1 evidence with expert clinical reasoning. Br J Sports Med 2015;49:923–34.

30. Female athlete issues for the team physician: a consensus statement—2017 update. Curr Sports Med Rep 2018;17(5):163–71.

31. AOSSM female athlete issues for the team physician: a consensus statement. Available at: https://www.sportsmed.org/AOSSMIMIS/members/downloads/education/ConsensusStatements/FemaleAthlete.pdf. Accessed December 11, 2018.

32. Available at: http://forms.acsm.org/tpc/PDFs/35%20Ireland.pdf. Accessed December 11, 2018.

33. Burnham JM, Wright V. Update on anterior cruciate ligament rupture and care in the female athlete. Clin Sports Med 2017;36(4):703–15.

34. Webner D. Knee injury (ligamentous). Essential evidence plus. Wiley; 2018.

35. Jarbo KA, Hartigan DE, Scott KL, et al. Accuracy of the lever sign test in the diagnosis of anterior cruciate ligament injuries. Orthop J Sports Med 2017;5(10). 2325967117729809.

36. Frobell RB, Roos EM, Roos HP, et al. A randomized trial of treatment for acute anterior cruciate ligament tears. N Engl J Med 2010;363(4):331–42.

37. Voskanian N. ACL Injury prevention in female athletes: review of the literature and practical considerations in implementing an ACL prevention program. Curr Rev Musculoskelet Med 2013;6(2):158–63.

38. Ireland ML. Anterior cruciate ligament injury in female athletes: epidemiology. J Athl Train 1999;34(2):150–4.

39. Thomas DT, Erdman KA, Burke LM. American College of Sports Medicine joint position statement. Nutrition and athletic performance. Med Sci Sports Exerc 2016;48(3):543–68 [Erratum: Med Sci Sports Exerc. 2017;49(1):222].

40. Petkus DL, Murray-Kolb LE, De Souza MJ. The unexplored crossroads of the female athlete triad and iron deficiency: a narrative review. Sports Med 2017;47(9): 1721–37.

41. Beard J, Tobin B. Iron status and exercise. Am J Clin Nutr 2000;72(2 Suppl): 594S–7S.

42. Pedlar CR, Brugnara C, Bruinvels G, et al. Iron balance and iron supplementation for the female athlete: a practical approach. Eur J Sport Sci 2018;18(2): 295–305.
43. Alaunyte I, Stojceska V, Plunkett A. Iron and the female athlete: a review of dietary treatment methods for improving iron status and exercise performance. J Int Soc Sports Nutr 2015;12:38.

Principles of Rehabilitation

Michelle Futrell, MA, ATC, SCAT[a],*, Susan L. Rozzi, PhD, ATC, SCAT[b]

KEYWORDS

- Rehabilitation • Tissue healing phases • Problem-based approach

KEY POINTS

- Developing and implementing a rehabilitation program requires a working knowledge of the pathologic condition of the injury, a firm grasp of the healing process, and a thorough appraisal of available treatment options.
- Seven overarching principles can be applied to any rehabilitation program: avoiding aggravation, timing, compliance, individualization, specific sequencing, intensity, and consideration of the total patient.
- Therapeutic exercises selected for inclusion in rehabilitation plans vary but typically incorporate exercises to address the following: range of motion; flexibility; muscle strength, endurance, and power; proprioception and neuromuscular control; cardiorespiratory fitness; and functional and sport-specific activities.
- A problem-based approach to creating and implementing a treatment plan takes a cyclical approach that requires the clinician to continually assess, identify problems to be addressed, screen treatment options, create goals, implement treatment plans, and reassess.

INTRODUCTION

Developing and implementing a rehabilitation program can be one of the most complex patient care skills to manage because it requires the ability to coordinate a working knowledge of the pathologic condition of the injury, a firm grasp of the healing process of the involved tissues, and a thorough appraisal of the available treatment options that is then combined with the creativity of the clinician and limited by the psychological approach and motivation of the patient. At its best, a thorough rehabilitation program is a coordinated effort of all members of a patient's health care team driven by a shared philosophy and desire to return the patient to preinjury status. Disconnects in any of the above areas can result in poor patient outcomes. Rehabilitation is unique in that many times innovations made in clinical practice drive changes to widely accepted treatment protocols that are later investigated as opposed to other

[a] Department of Health and Human Performance, Center for Academic Performance & Persistence, College of Charleston, 66 George Street, Charleston, SC29424, USA; [b] Department of Health and Human Performance, College of Charleston, 66 George Street, Charleston, SC 29424, USA
* Corresponding author.
E-mail address: FutrellM@cofc.edu

Prim Care Clin Office Pract 47 (2020) 87–103
https://doi.org/10.1016/j.pop.2019.10.004
0095-4543/20/© 2019 Elsevier Inc. All rights reserved.
primarycare.theclinics.com

aspects of medicine in which research and measured patient outcomes drive changes to clinical practice.[1] A prime example of this would be the development of the accelerated rehabilitation protocol following anterior cruciate ligament reconstruction. Rehabilitation is also unique in that although various protocols exist that provide normative guidelines for progression, individual patient differences will always necessitate a constant need for clinicians to ensure that the right treatment is being prescribed to the right patient at the right time to achieve the best outcomes. For these reasons, it is important that clinicians consistently evaluate best practices and weigh the available evidence to develop patient-specific rehabilitation plans. In this article, a conceptual framework is provided to guide clinicians through the decision-making process for identifying and selecting appropriate treatment options when developing a rehabilitation protocol. This conceptual framework was developed because patients are unique, and their injuries respond in different ways. It is important for clinicians to approach rehabilitation from the mindset of repeatedly evaluating the patient, considering treatment options, and adjusting and adapting treatments. After presenting this conceptual framework it will be applied to 3 different injuries at different phases in the rehabilitation process to provide examples of the conceptual framework in practice.

PRINCIPLES OF REHABILITATION

Each rehabilitation program is unique, but there are key (overarching) principles that should be considered when developing a rehabilitation program.[2] Houglum[2] identifies 7 general principles that form the foundation on which a rehabilitation program is built and can be applied to any rehabilitation program (**Box 1**).[2]

- Avoid aggravation: Care should be taken when exercises are prescribed and progressed so as not to aggravate the injury. The injured tissue should be observed to determine response to imposed loads, and the patient should be monitored during exercise bouts whenever possible for coordinated movement and confidence with the injured tissue.
- Timing: Rehabilitation should begin as soon as tolerated by the healing tissue in order to minimize the deleterious impacts of rest and immobilization. Delays in initiating rehabilitation will result in a delayed recovery process.
- Compliance: Adherence to prescribed exercises and completing exercises correctly and at an appropriate intensity are important to a successful

---

Box 1
Principles of rehabilitation

Basic rehabilitation principles

- Avoid aggravation
- Timing
- Compliance
- Individualization
- Specific sequencing
- Intensity
- Total patient

Data from Houglum PA. Therapeutic exercise for musculoskeletal injuries. 4th edition. Champaign, IL: Human Kinetics; 2016.

rehabilitation program. Helping patients understand the scope and trajectory of the rehabilitation program often increases compliance.

- Individualization: Rehabilitation protocols may be used as guidelines, but each patient will respond differently, and the program should be progressed based on individual response. Some of the factors that will contribute to individual patient progression may include, but are not limited to, history of previous injury, severity of the injury, level of motivation, available support systems, injury complications, and internal or external pressures.
- Specific sequencing: Sequencing in the rehabilitation process should be based on the severity of the injury, the physiologic processes occurring during the various phases of healing, and the response of the injured tissues to imposed demands. Each type of exercise in a rehabilitation program should be intentionally introduced and progressed with these factors in mind.
- Intensity: Intensity of the rehabilitation program should be closely monitored to ensure that the healing tissues are subjected to forces that encourage overload and challenge the patient without disrupting the healing process or negatively impacting patient motivation and compliance.
- Total patient: Although a rehabilitation program will focus on a specific injured tissue, care should be taken to minimize impact on overall fitness and conditioning levels. Deconditioning is always an inherent risk associated with any type of injury. In order to be prepared to return to activity, conditioning of uninvolved tissues and systems must be maximized.

COMPONENTS OF A REHABILITATION PLAN

The components selected for inclusion in a rehabilitation plan will vary based on the pathologic condition and the individual patient needs and in most cases are limited only by the creativity of the rehabilitation professional. However, the following components should be considered for inclusion when appropriate (**Box 2**):

1. Range of motion: A full unrestricted range of motion is necessary to achieve full function. A variety of factors may contribute to range-of-motion limitations, including pain, swelling, scar tissue, adhesions, foreign bodies, joint hypomobility, inflexibility of muscles crossing the joint, and lack of muscle strength. Rehabilitation programs that stress early motion and weight-bearing demonstrate better outcomes.[3]
2. Flexibility: Maximizing flexibility of muscles crossing joints can minimize the impact that tight musculature may have on joint motion. Flexibility deficits are best

---

Box 2
Components of a rehabilitation plan

Rehabilitation plan components

- Range of motion
- Flexibility
- Muscular strength, endurance, and power
- Proprioception and neuromuscular control
- Cardiorespiratory endurance
- Functional progressions

managed through the use of various stretching techniques using static, dynamic, and proprioceptive neuromuscular facilitation stretching principles.

3. Muscular strength, endurance, and power: In order to provide support and stability and to promote motion, muscles must be able to exert force against resistance. In addition, muscles must have the capacity to contract repeatedly for an extended period of time. In many athletic activities, muscles must also be able to generate power. Power is defined as the ability to exert force against resistance in a very short time period.[4] Muscular strength, endurance, and power can be trained through isometric, progressive resistive, isokinetic, and plyometric exercises.

4. Proprioception and neuromuscular control: The recovery of balance, coordination, and agility is essential for restoring preinjury level coordinated movements in multiple planes needed for full function and to minimize risk of injury or reinjury. Exercises to train proprioception, balance, and agility should be incorporated throughout the rehabilitation program.

5. Cardiorespiratory endurance: A coordinated effort of the heart and lungs is necessary to support work associated with exercise and activities of daily living. Injury can result in a deconditioning response in as little as 2 to 4 weeks. This is demonstrated by decreases in Vo_{2max}, blood volume, and stroke volume and increases in resting heart rate.[5–7] Including cardiorespiratory training exercises throughout the rehabilitation process allows maintenance of fitness levels, which will promote a more seamless return to full activity.

6. Functional progressions: After range of motion and strength deficits have been addressed, and the patient has developed sufficient proprioception and neuromuscular control, functional and sports-specific activities in a controlled environment can be infused into the patient's rehabilitation program. In this way, healing tissues will be exposed to the forces associated with the activities in which the patient participates and provide an opportunity to adapt and regain coordinated movement and skills.

CONCEPTUAL MODEL OF PROBLEM-BASED APPROACH TO REHABILITATION

Because there are so many variables that come into play when designing a rehabilitation program, it is helpful to have a decision-making scheme that can be applied to each individual situation and modified appropriately for each patient. The conceptual model presented draws on a cyclical problem-solving approach to clinical practice that requires the clinician to continually assess, identify problems to be addressed, screen treatment options, create goals, implement treatment plans, and reassess progress (**Fig. 1**).[8] This process is then repeated at the beginning of each phase of the rehabilitation process and within a phase as interim goals are met. The following section explains the conceptual model of a problem-based approach to rehabilitation.

1. Identification of problems: The initial step in the process is to identify the patient's key problems. Through a comprehensive medical history, the clinician can identify the patient's chief complaint while also carefully considering any pertinent information that may impact the treatment and rehabilitation process. In addition to the medical history, an initial physical examination provides the foundational information that will be used in the program development and goal-setting process.[9] After completion of the examination, the clinician should be able to create a problem list from all the abnormal findings. Each problem is a potential contributor to the patient's dysfunction and serves as the basis for the creation of treatment goals.[9] This process will be repeated at various intervals throughout the treatment process.

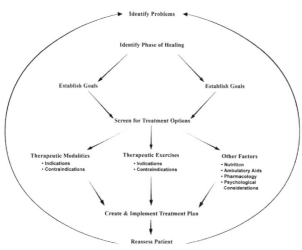

Fig. 1. Conceptual model of problem-based approach to rehabilitation.

2. Identify tissue healing phase: It is very important to consider where the injured tissues fall in the continuum of the healing process. It is also important to note that selection of appropriate treatment options relies heavily on enhancing and supporting the physiologic healing process and protecting the injured tissues as they heal. Failure to recognize this can often result in a delay in healing and poor rehabilitation outcomes. Delayed healing often results in a chronic inflammatory process that impacts progression of rehabilitation. Healing is impacted by both local and systemic factors. Some local factors include oxygenation, infection, presence of foreign bodies, edema, venous insufficiency, hypertrophic scarring, muscle spasm, and muscle atrophy, whereas systemic factors include age, sex-related hormones, stress, chronic medical conditions, medications, obesity, alcohol consumption, smoking, nutrition, and humidity (**Box 3**).[2,4,8,10]

3. Establish treatment goals: Goals provide structure on which a treatment plan can be built and assist in the sequencing of the selected therapeutic interventions. In

Box 3
Factors impacting the healing process

Local Factors	Systemic Factors
Oxygenation	Age
Infection	Sex-related hormones
Foreign bodies	Stress
Hemorrhage	Chronic medical conditions (ie, diabetes, human immunodeficiency virus,
Edema	endocrine diseases, arthritis, carcinoma, autoimmune diseases)
Wound size	Medications (ie, antibiotics, antineoplastic, heparin, nicotine,
Venous	corticosteroids)
insufficiency	Obesity
Hypertrophic	Alcohol consumption
scarring	Smoking
Muscle spasm	Nutrition
Muscle atrophy	Humidity/climate

Data from Refs.[2,4,8,10]

addition, goals provide benchmarks to assess treatment efficacy. Each rehabilitation program will have both long-term and short-term treatment goals. Long-term goals are more comprehensive in nature and may require weeks or even months to accomplish. Long-term goals focus on end results of a treatment plan, and therefore, interim or short-term goals relate more specifically to performance objectives that can be accomplished within 2 weeks. Regardless of the type of goal, it should be functional in nature and include objective criteria that can be measured and reproduced.[11] Kettenbach[11] identifies key components of functional treatment goals as "audience, behavior, condition, degree, and timeframe." These components address the target of the goal, which is usually the patient, what will be achieved, how it will be measured, the standard required to meet the goal, and the time needed to meet the goal. This format is similar to the commonly used SMART goal format, which requires a goal to be specific (what will be achieved), measurable (how success is will be assessed), achievable (level required to meet the goal), relevant (has meaning for the participant and has necessary supports), and time framed (time in which the goal will be achieved).[12] Whenever possible, the patient should be involved in the goal-setting process because active involvement improves compliance with rehabilitation programs. Regardless of the approach, well-written goals are characterized by clearly measurable outcomes that leave no question as to whether the goal has been met. For example, if a patient's identified problem is unilateral limited knee flexion, then 1 short-term goal may read as follows: increase right knee flexion, measured in prone position using a standard goniometer, from 90° to 110°, in 14 days.

4. Screen for treatment options: Once goals have been identified, they must then be prioritized and compared with available therapeutic modalities and therapeutic exercise techniques. Key information to be considered when screening treatment options includes the type of tissues involved and the approximate depth of tissues of concern, type of pathologic condition, phase of healing, and anticipated forces and types of activities necessary for return to full activity.[8] Contraindicated therapeutic modalities and inappropriate therapeutic exercise program components can be eliminated. From the treatment options that remain, the clinician can then select those that are most appropriate for meeting the identified goals. Using the goal stated earlier of increasing right knee flexion, measured in prone position using a standard goniometer, from 90° to 110°, in 14 days the treatment options to address this goal may include cryotherapy, thermotherapy, manual therapies, active and passive stretching, joint mobilization, electrical stimulation, and strengthening exercises.

5. Establish and implement treatment plan: After identifying the patient's problems, identifying the healing phase of the tissues, setting treatment goals, and screening all available treatment options, a comprehensive treatment plan can then be established by selecting a combination of therapeutic modalities and exercises that address each of the goals identified in the previous step. Considering the treatment goals of increasing right knee flexion, measured in the prone position using a standard goniometer, from 90° to 110°, in 14 days, the treatment may include warm whirlpool or heat packs, massage or soft tissue mobilization, patellofemoral joint mobilization (inferior and superior patellar glides), tibiofemoral joint mobilization (distraction, posterior tibial glides), strengthening of the knee flexor muscles though a progressive resistive exercise program, and prolonged passive stretching and active stretching of the knee extensor muscles. This process of selecting treatments applies to each of the preestablished short-term and long-term treatment goals. A comprehensive treatment plan may also include means of addressing

other needs, including ambulatory aids like crutches, canes, or walking boots, pharmacologic treatment, such as over-the-counter analgesic medications, nutritional counseling to maximize healing or address body weight issues, and counseling to address the patient's identified psychological needs.

6. Reassess: Serial reevaluations will need to be conducted throughout the rehabilitation process to evaluate the effectiveness of the treatment provided and progress the treatment plan. These reevaluations should include both subjective and objective information that can then be used to modify short-term goals. Previously identified problems should be reevaluated, and short- and long-term goals should be assessed to determine the effectiveness of the treatment program. Validated subjective or objective outcome measures may also be used to monitor progress. To be effective, care should be taken to select an outcome measure that is patient specific, region specific, and disease specific whenever possible.[13] New problems may also be identified during the reassessment process. All available treatment options should also be reassessed because techniques that may have been contraindicated early in the rehabilitation progression may now be available for use. Case in point, when a patient progresses from the inflammatory to regeneration phase of rehabilitation, increased tissue temperature is no longer contraindicated so continuous ultrasounds, moist hot pack, warm whirlpool, and shortwave diathermy can now to be added to the list of available therapeutic modalities to be considered. New goals can be set, and the treatment plan can then be modified and progressed. The process continues on a cyclical basis until all goals have been met, and the patient returns to preinjury status. When specific, measurable, and functional goals are linked to problems identified during the evaluative process, and those goals are connected to well-thought-out therapeutic interventions, a comprehensive rehabilitation program will result (see **Fig. 1**).[8,9]

APPLICATION OF THE PROBLEM-BASED APPROACH TO REHABILITATION

The following 3 diagrams and their associated explanations illustrate how the problem-based approach to rehabilitation, as presented in the conceptual model, can be applied to musculoskeletal conditions in differing phases of the tissue-healing process, and thus with differing problems to be addressed in the rehabilitation program (**Table 1**). Condition1: Acute Hamstring Strain in the Acute injury and Inflammatory phase (**Fig. 2**); Condition 2: Ulnar Collateral Ligament Sprain in the Motion Phase (**Fig. 3**), Condition 3: Lateral Ankle Sprain in the Strength/Function Phase (**Fig. 4**). Note that because each condition is in a different phase of the healing process, identified problems, associated short-term and long-term treatment goals, and available therapeutic modalities and exercises are individualized.

CONDITION 1: ACUTE HAMSTRING INJURY IN THE ACUTE INJURY AND INFLAMMATORY PHASES

The acute injury phase of the rehabilitation process begins as soon as the tissue is injured. As a response to tissue damage, the physiologic healing process is initiated. Initial evaluation at the point of injury provides key information about the nature of the injury and the suspected pathologic condition. The most accurate physical examination of soft tissue structures and particularly ligament laxity occurs before the onset of inflammation. It is in this phase that initial diagnostic tests may be ordered to confirm physical findings and guide treatment. The applied model of this injury is explained in later discussion and presented in **Fig. 2**.

Futrell & Rozzi

Table 1
Summary of applied model of problem-based approach to rehabilitation

Phase	Tissue Healing	Goals	Therapeutic Modalities	Therapeutic Exercise	Other Factors
Acute Injury Phase (0-3 d)					
Problems: Pain Swelling Loss of function	Acute inflammation Vasoconstriction followed by vasodilation Clot is produced Blood and fluid accumulation	Promote clot formation Protect healing tissues Modulate pain Minimize swelling accumulation	Ice Compression Estim Ultrasound laser	Rest Elevation	Nutrition Ambulatory aids Protective aids
Inflammatory Phase (1 d to 3 d)					
Problems: Pain Swelling Spasm Edema Decreased function	Inflammation Phagocytosis Lattice-like matrix is created	Promote clot formation Protect healing tissues Modulate pain Minimize swelling/edema accumulation	Cryotherapy Compression Elevation Estim Ultrasound	Nothing to disrupt the clot Exercise uninvolved area Gentle range of motion (ROM)	Nutrition Pharmacology Ambulatory aids
Motion Phase (3 d to 7 d)					
Problems: Edema Decreased ROM Strength deficits Loss of function	Repair/regeneration Angiogenesis Collagen proliferation	Reduce edema Regain ROM Protect scar formation Initiate muscle reeducation Maintain cardiorespiratory endurance Improve flexibility Progressive weight-bearing or functional skills	Cryotherapy progressing to thermotherapy Estim: interferential, Russian/HiVolt (muscle reeducation) Ultrasound Joint mobilizations Massage Intermittent compression	ROM; (PROM-AAROM, AROM) Strength; isometrics Flexibility Cardio	Nutrition Pharmacology

Strength & Function Phase (5 d to 24 mo)

Problems:	Remodeling	Goals:	Thermotherapy	Flexibility Exs	Nutrition
Tensile strength of injured tissue	Wound reorganizes Type III collagen replaced with aligned type I collagen	Increase circulation	Estim: muscle reeducation	PRE	Pharmacology
Strength and power deficits		Promote scar realignment	Ultrasound	Isokinetics	Taping & bracing
Muscle atrophy		Regain full ROM	Joint mobilizations	NM coordination	Psychological factors
Decreased ROM		Gain muscular strength		Balance	
Lack of full flexibility		Improve NM control and coordinator		Proprioception	
Decreased NM control, balance, coordination, and agility		Progress functional activities		Agility	
		Maintain CV condition		Plyometrics	
				Functional activities	
				Cardiovasular activities	

Abbreviations: AAROM, Active Assistive Range of Motion; AROM, Active Range of Motion; Cardio, Cardiovascular Exercise; CR, Cardiorespiratory; CV, Cardiovascular; Exs, Exercises; NM, Neuromuscular; PROM, Passive Range of Motion; ROM-Range of Motion.

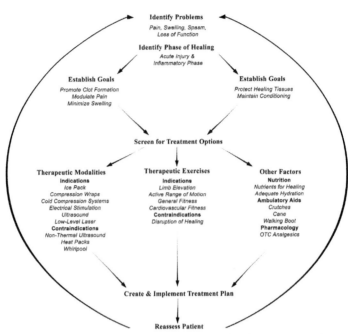

Fig. 2. Applied model of problem-based approach to rehabilitation: acute hamstring strain in acute injury and inflammatory phase. OTC, over-the-counter.

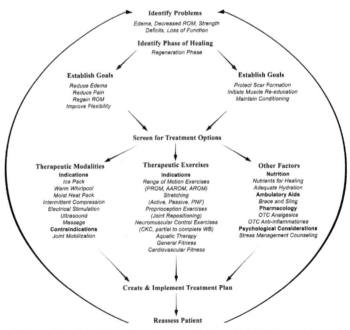

Fig. 3. Applied model of problem-based approach to rehabilitation: ulnar collateral ligament sprain in motion phase. CKC, closed kinetic chain; PNF, proprioceptive neuromuscular facilitation; WB, weight bearing.

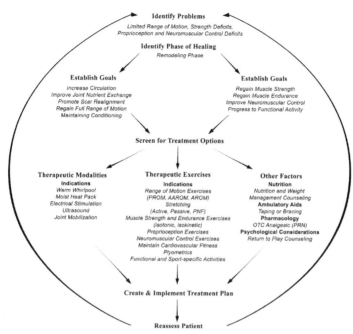

Fig. 4. Applied model of problem-based approach to rehabilitation: lateral ankle sprain in strength/function phase.

Acute Injury Phase (Time of Injury to 3 Days)

Problems

For most patients, the primary complaints in this phase include pain, swelling, and loss of function. It is often these problems that prompt a patient to seek evaluation.

Tissue healing

The acute inflammatory phase of the healing process is often referred to as hemostasis. In this phase, damage to the tissue secondary to the forces applied also results in damage to the local vasculature. This tissue damage is responsible for initiating the healing process. As a result of bleeding associated with vessel damage, an immediate vasoconstriction occurs, followed by a reflex vasodilation secondary to the hypoxic environment that is created. Platelets and other chemical mediators aggregate at the site and produce a platelet plug. As a result, blood and other lymphatic fluids begin to accumulate in the area.[2,4,8,14,15]

Goals

Based on the common problems identified in this phase of rehabilitation, common goals would include the following: promoting clot formation, protecting healing tissues, modulating pain, and minimizing accumulation of swelling.

Screen treatment options

Therapeutic modalities that should be considered in this phase include the following: ice, compression, electrical stimulation (interferential, premodulated), ultrasound (pulsed), and laser. Protected rest and elevation of the injured tissues are the primary therapeutic exercise and treatment options in this phase.[2,8,9]

Other factors

Ambulatory aids, such as crutches, canes, or walking boots, should be considered for lower-extremity injuries, or protective supports, such as slings, braces, splints, or immobilizers, should also be considered to protect the healing tissues from excessive motion. In this phase, patients often experience a negative emotional response, especially if the injury is severe in nature. Patients most often seek to manage these emotions by reaching out to family, friends, and teammates for social support.[16]

Inflammatory Phase (1 Day to 3 Days)

As the first hours following injury pass, the injury enters the inflammatory phase of rehabilitation, and with it adjustments to treatment options should occur.

Problems

In this phase of the rehabilitation process, key problems include continued pain, swelling, and loss of function. Pain, loss of function, and reflexive splinting to protect injured tissues may also lead to muscle spasm. In addition, fluid collecting in the intercellular spaces as well as by-products of inflammation lead to edema.

Tissue healing

The inflammatory phase of the healing process centers on clearing the injured area of waste products. Neutrophils promote phagocytosis to clear cells that might promote chronic inflammation if allowed to linger in the area. Fibroblasts also begin to lay down the extracellular matrix on which the scar will be built.[14,15,17]

Goals

Goals in this phase again focus on protecting the healing tissues. Because a scar has not yet been formed, it is important that healing tissues not be subjected to forces that might disrupt the injured tissues or cause additional inflammation because phagocytes are working to clear the area. Steps should be taken to promote an environment conducive to clot formation while also modulating pain and minimizing swelling and accumulation of edema. The more fluid accumulation is controlled, the more quickly range of motion and function can be restored.

Screen treatment options

Therapeutic modalities that should be considered in this phase include modalities that do not create an increase in tissue temperature like cryotherapy and nonthermal ultrasound. For pain control, electrical stimulation should be considered and can be combined with cryotherapy. Continued use of elevation and compression to minimize accumulation of edema should also be considered. Therapeutic exercise of injured tissues should be minimized so as not to disrupt clot formation. Gentle pain-free range-of-motion exercises may be initiated while avoiding motions that stress the injured tissue because muscle contraction may also promote edema reduction. Exercise of uninvolved areas can be considered to minimize impacts of lack of activity.[2,8,9]

Other factors

Similar to the acute injury phase, ambulatory aids or protective devices may be indicated to protect the injured tissues. Patients will continue to seek social support and may begin to question the nature of the injury and what the rehabilitation plan may entail.[16] In addition, ensuring adequate nutrient consumption to create the best healing environment remains a valid concern. In this stage of healing, adequate protein is necessary for enzyme synthesis and to promote cell proliferation and collagen formation. In addition, the amino acid glutamine plays a role in stimulating the inflammatory response, and essential fatty acids are used in prostaglandin synthesis.[17] Vitamin A plays a critical role in the inflammatory process because it stimulates macrophage production. Once the acute injury phase has passed and the inflammatory phase has started, anti-inflammatory medications may be considered to manage pain and minimize excessive production of the by-products of inflammation.

CONDITION 2: ULNAR COLLATERAL LIGAMENT SPRAIN IN THE MOTION PHASE
Motion Phase (3 Days to 7 Days)

In the motion phase of the rehabilitation process, the impacts of inflammation must be addressed. The problems identified in this phase may become more apparent as time passes, the pain of the initial injury decreases, and the patient begins to test the injured tissue. **Fig. 3** illustrates the application of the problem-based approach to an injury in the motion phase.

Problems

Edema commonly results from the inflammatory process and with it an associated decrease in range of motion. Strength deficits may also be apparent because of muscle inhibition secondary to edema formation and because the healing tissue is not yet stabilized. As a result of each of those problems, functional deficits also continue.

Tissue healing

This phase of healing is characterized by tissue repair and regeneration. Once the injured tissue is successfully marginalized and cleared of waste products, tissue regeneration can begin. Angiogenesis occurs first as preexisting vessels grow into the area.[17] Adequate oxygen supply during this phase of healing is necessary for a positive outcome because metabolic activity is increased and relies heavily on oxygen availability. Fibroblasts then accumulate along the vessels and begin to produce collagen and elastin to fill in the extracellular matrix that forms the structure of the scar.[15]

Goals

Goals in the motion phase center on managing the impact of the inflammatory process and providing controlled forces to protect the scar as it forms. Reducing edema and regaining range of motion are important for the patient to be able to progress to the next phases of rehabilitation. Flexibility exercises for the surrounding musculature may also support increases in range of motion. Muscle reeducation should also be initiated and can be completed in a limited range if necessary, through the use of isometric contractions.

Screen treatment options

In this phase, therapeutic modalities can be progressed from cryotherapy to thermotherapy as point tenderness decreases and the scar begins to provide some stability to the injured area. However, cryotherapy may also be indicated after treatment to minimize any inflammation caused by the treatment. Electrical stimulation should be considered using muscle reeducation parameters and pain control parameters after treatment as needed. Joint mobilizations may be used to promote joint arthrokinematics. To remove edema, massage, intermittent compression, and ultrasound can be considered. Ultrasound may also be used to enhance healing. In combination with modalities, range-of-motion and flexibility exercises should be used to facilitate full unrestricted motion. Passive range-of-motion and active-assisted range-of-motion exercises will allow motion without requiring excessive forces until strength and stability will support active range of motion. As muscle reeducation exercises are initiated, isometrics should be added first because they will allow strength gains without requiring full motion. Cardiorespiratory endurance should be maintained by selecting a training method that does not stress the injured tissue. For example, a recumbent bicycle can be used if the patient is unable to run comfortably or if weight bearing is contraindicated. As pain and function allows, weight bearing and functional skills can also be initiated.[2,8,9]

Other factors

As the rehabilitation process progresses, patient questioning of the rehabilitation plan may increase as will the frustration associated with the injury. Patients may begin to turn toward their care provider for support and encouragement to manage the emotional aspects of the injury.[16] It is important that in both the motion and the strength/function phases that adequate caloric intake is available to support the increased metabolic processes associated with wound healing. Guidelines from the American Society for Parenteral and Enteral Nutrition and the Wound Healing Society recommend 30 to 35 kcal/kg/d, which is considered to be optimal intake to support wound healing.[17,18] The primary energy source for collagen synthesis and wound healing comes from glucose. In addition, all stages of wound healing require adequate protein intake to enhance collagen synthesis and rate of wound healing. Vitamin A and C play important roles in this phase of healing because they stimulate capillary formation and contribute to collagen synthesis.

CONDITION 3: LATERAL ANKLE SPRAIN IN THE STRENGTH/FUNCTION PHASE
Strength/Function Phase (5 Days to 24 Months)

The final phase of the rehabilitation process is the strength/function phase. This phase is the longest and is highlighted by progressively increasing strength and stability of the injured tissues and a focus on moving toward functional and sport-specific activities in preparation for discharge. Depending on the severity of the injury and length of the total rehabilitation process, this phase may be approached by subdividing into an early phase that focuses on strength and stability and a late phase targeted at functional skills.[2] The applied model for this phase can be found in **Fig. 4**.

Problems

In this phase, the healing tissue still lacks tensile strength. In addition, strength and power deficits of surrounding musculature persist, and depending on the length of immobilization, muscle atrophy may also be a concern. Although range of motion should be returning, full motion may not be achieved until sometime during this phase. Flexibility of surrounding musculature should remain a focus because movement toward functional activities will require full, unrestricted motion of the involved joints. Assessment of functional components, such as neuromuscular control, balance, coordination, and agility, will be important to measure because these are necessary to progress to return to full function and discharge.

Tissue healing

This phase of healing is highlighted by remodeling and realignment of the healing tissue. Initially, fibroblasts fill in the collagen matrix that was created in the regeneration phase with type III collagen. As compared with uninjured tissue, type III collagen makes up about 30% of the scar tissue as compared with 10% to 20% in its uninjured counterpart. Increased collagen formation takes place for 4 to 5 weeks as the wound gradually increases in size and strength. At approximately the 3-week mark, the strength of the healing tissues is approximately 20% of uninjured tissue.[17] When the scar reaches adequate size and strength, type III collagen is gradually replaced with type I collagen. As type I collagen is produced, it is also realigned along the lines of force to which the healing tissue is subjected. This principle is known as Wolff Law and was first identified in 1892 by James Wolff, who identified that providing small mechanical loads to healing bone prompted new tissue formation and decreased the removal of too much callus as was seen when load was removed.[19] This principle speaks to the importance of providing intentionally selected and controlled forces to healing tissue during the rehabilitation process. It is also important to note that as the ratio of type III to type I collagen decreases approximately 6 weeks into the healing process, an associated decrease in tensile strength of the healing tissue may occur. Additional care should be taken by clinicians to provide controlled forces to reduce the risk of reinjury.[15]

Goals
In the strength/function phase, patient goals center on promoting scar realignment through provision of controlled forces. Regaining full range of motion and muscular strength is the primary focus of the early portion of this phase because those are necessary for initiation of functional activities. Once range of motion and strength are achieved, goals shift toward regaining functional skills in the late stages of this phase. Functional skills include reestablishing neuromuscular control, coordination, balance, agility, and power. Finally, sport- or activity-specific exercises should be broken down by intensity and degree of difficulty so they can be gradually incorporated into the rehabilitation plan. Throughout this phase, cardiorespiratory endurance and flexibility should also be maintained.

Screen treatment options
In this phase of rehabilitation, most therapeutic modalities are not contraindicated. Clinicians should assess the specific indications and physiologic responses provided by each therapeutic modality to best align with the specific goal to be met. Thermotherapy and ultrasound to promote tissue temperature increases and enhanced circulation and nutrition as well as electrical stimulation with a focus on muscle reeducation may be indicated. If joint motion remains restricted, joint mobilization techniques should be considered. As the tissue becomes stronger and more stable, continued use of a variety of strengthening exercises should be included focusing on progressive resistive exercises and isokinetics to introduce continual resistance at varying speeds. Later in this phase, exercises should be introduced to establish a baseline for functional activities. These exercises would include balance, proprioception, and neuromuscular control exercises. Plyometric exercises, high-intensity jumping and landing exercises that focus on maximizing the stretch reflex, can be used to regain speed, power, and efficiency of movement before initiation of functional progressions. The purpose of a functional progression is to retrain the skills necessary for full return to activity. These skills are presented in a logical progression that gradually increases in difficulty and intensity. A functional progression for a patient recovering from a lateral ankle sprain would begin with jogging followed by jogging in a figure-8 pattern, progressing to a Z pattern, to cutting on command. Once those skills are mastered, the speed at which the exercises are completed can be increased. Skipping, jumping, and hopping might also be included depending on the nature of activity to which the patient needs to return. Throughout this phase, cardiorespiratory endurance should also be maintained in a manner and can be trained during functional exercises as well.[2,4,8,9]

Other factors Protein intake is critical to collagen synthesis, and protein deficits impact the strength of the healing tissue. Protein supplementation may need to be considered for older adults because inactivity can result in sarcopenia and decreased immune system function.[17] Recommended Dietary Reference Intake for protein is

0.8 g/kg/d but may be increased to 1.25 to 1.5 g/kg/d during the wound-healing process, especially in nonhealing or chronic wounds. In addition to macronutrients, patients should increase intake of whole foods high in micronutrients that support wound healing, collagen formation, and tissue growth, including magnesium, copper, and zinc.[17] During the late stages of the strength/function phase, patients will be progressed back to functional activities. Taping and bracing may be considered to provide additional support and proprioceptive feedback. As the rehabilitation program progresses, patients will often demonstrate a more cautious approach because they may be anxious about reinjury and how the injured limb will respond to increased demands. Functional progressions may serve to decrease this anxiety and increase the patient's excitement about return to full activity and discharge.[16]

RETURN TO ACTIVITY CONSIDERATIONS

Return to activity criteria are a critical piece in the management of all injuries but are rarely standardized and may oftentimes be influenced by persons who are not trained in a medical decision-making process. Therefore, clinicians may want to consider using a decision-based return to play model outlined by Creighton and colleagues[20] that includes the following:

1. Evaluation of health status, including signs, symptoms, medical history, and functional testing
2. Evaluation of participation risk, including sport, position, level of competition, and ability to protect the injured structure
3. Decision modification factors, including timing, internal and external pressure, conflicts of interest, and litigation potential

Other key factors that should be considered when reaching the decision to release the patient to return to limited or full participation are status of the healing process, full unrestricted range of motion, strength equal to that of the bilateral limb, adequate neuromuscular control and proprioceptive protective mechanism, and appropriate cardiorespiratory fitness levels.[2,21] In the final stages of the rehabilitation process, functional progressions and functional testing provide clinicians with the opportunity to assess the patient's ability to demonstrate activity-specific skills at full speed as well as full confidence in the injured limb. Before return, the clinician should discuss any potential risks with return to play, provide instructions and recommendations for continued rehabilitation, and assess the patient's psychological readiness to return to activity.[2,22]

DISCLOSURE

The authors have no financial or other associations with companies related to this article, topic and content.

REFERENCES

1. Sauers EL, Snyder AR. A team approach: demonstrating sport rehabilitation effectiveness and enhancing patient care through clinical outcomes assessment. J Sport Rehabil 2011;20(1):3–7.
2. Houglum PA. Therapeutic exercise for musculoskeletal injuries. 4th edition. Champaign (IL): Human Kinetics; 2016.
3. Millett PJ, Wickiewicz TI, Warren RF. Current concepts. Motion loss after ligament injuries to the knee: part I: causes. Am J Sports Med 2001;29(5):664–75.

4. Prentice WE. Principles of athletic training. A guide to evidence-based clinical practice. 16th edition. New York: McGraw Hill; 2017.
5. Cardoza MA, Gonzalez-Badillo M, Gonzalez-Badillo J. In-season resistance training and detraining in professional team handball players. J Strength Cond Res 2006;20(3):563–71.
6. Costill D, Fink WJ, Hargreves M, et al. Metabolic characteristics of skeletal muscle during detraining from competitive swimming. Med Sci Sports Exerc 1985; 17(3):339–43.
7. Coyle E, Martin S, Bloomfield O, et al. Effects of detraining on responses to submaximal exercise. J Appl Physiol (1985) 1985;59:853–9.
8. Starkey C. Therapeutic modalities. 3rd edition. Philadelphia: FA Davis; 2004.
9. Higgins M. Therapeutic exercise. From theory to practice. Philadelphia: FA Davis Company; 2011.
10. Guo S, Dipietro LA. Factors affecting wound healing. J Dent Res 2010;89(3): 219–29.
11. Kettenbach G. Writing SOAP notes. 3rd edition. Philadelphia: FA Davis; 2004.
12. Bovend'Eerdt TJ, Botell RE, Wade DT. Writing SMART rehabilitation goals and achieving goal attainment scaling: a practical guide. Clin Rehabil 2009;23(4): 352–61.
13. Martin RL, Irrgang JJ. A survey of self-reported outcome instruments for the foot and ankle. J Orthop Sports Phys Ther 2007;37(2):72–84.
14. Diegelmann RF, Evans MC. Wound healing: an overview of acute, fibrotic, and delayed healing. Front Biosci 2004;9:283–9.
15. Janis HE, Harrison B. Wound healing part I: basic science. Plast Reconstr Surg 2016;138(3S):9s–17s.
16. Clement D, Arvinen-Barrow M, Fetty T. Psychosocial responses during different phases of sport-injury rehabilitation: a qualitative study. J Athl Train 2015;50(1): 95–104.
17. Stechmiller JK. Understanding the role of nutrition and wound healing. Nutr Clin Pract 2010;25(1):61–8.
18. Stechmiller JK, Cowan L, Johns P. Nutrition and wound healing. In: Gottschlich M, DeLegge MH, Mattox T, et al, editors. The A.S.P.E.N. Nutrition Support Science Core Curriculum: a case-based approach—the adult patient. Dubuque (IA): Kendall Hunt; 2007. p. 405–23.
19. Frost HM. A 2003 update of bone physiology and Wolff's Law for clinicians. Angle Orthod 2004;74(1):3–15.
20. Creighton DW, Shrier I, Shultz R, et al. Return-to-play in sport: a decision-based model. Clin J Sport Med 2010;20(5):379–85.
21. Herring SA, Kibler WB, Putulian M. The team physician and the return-to-play decision: a consensus statement–2012 update. Med Sci Sports Exerc 2012;44(12): 2446–8.
22. Clover J, Wall J. Return-to-play criteria following sports injury. Clin Sports Med 2010;29(1):169–75.

Common Upper-Extremity Injuries

Alexei DeCastro, MD

KEYWORDS

- Athletes • Sports medicine • Tennis • Upper-extremity injuries • Shoulder injuries
- Hand and wrist injuries

KEY POINTS

- Upper-extremity injuries are very common in both sports and regular physical activities; therefore, it is important to take into consideration specific aspects of the types of sports or activities of the athlete.
- Injuries to the rotator cuff are a very common source for dysfunction in athletes in all sports and at all levels of competition. Management of rotator cuff injuries is guided by the type of injury and severity and is initially treated either conservatively or surgically, and based on the patient's age, size of and location of the tear, and activity limitations.
- Overuse injuries of the elbow and forearm are very common in athletes. Pain may come from within the joint or the surrounding soft tissue structures, such as the medial and lateral epicondyles.
- Wrist pain often can be a challenging presenting injury to patients and athletes. It can be classified as acute pain caused by a trauma or as subacute/chronic pain. Acute wrist pain can be caused by conditions such as contusions, fractures, ligament sprains, and instability. Chronic pain usually results from overuse or may be a caused by previous injury.
- The fingers are the part of the upper extremity used for touch, feel, fine-motor skills, and performance of activities of daily living. Finger and metacarpal fractures are reportedly the most common sports-related fractures and are commonly seen in the office. Most, if recognized and diagnosed properly, can be managed appropriately, do not threaten limb viability, long-term function, and even can return to play. These finger injuries are most important to catch and diagnose because the greatest morbidity from these injuries would be from a delay in diagnosis or missed injuries deformity, which affect function.

INTRODUCTION

Upper-extremity injuries are very common in both sports and regular physical activities; therefore, it is important to take into consideration specific aspects of the types of sports or activities of the athlete. Treating providers need to know the physiopathology of these injuries in greater detail in order to achieve the best possible

Department of Family Medicine, Medical University of South Carolina, 5 Charleston Center, Charleston, SC 29401, USA
E-mail address: decastroa@musc.edu

Prim Care Clin Office Pract 47 (2020) 105–114
https://doi.org/10.1016/j.pop.2019.10.005
0095-4543/20/© 2019 Elsevier Inc. All rights reserved.

treatment. However, some injuries may appear relatively benign, but require prompt referral for surgical management. The main focus is on specific diagnoses and physiopathology, which are important factors for understanding treatment strategies. Specific treatments introduced more recently will also be mentioned, focusing particularly on treatments for tendinopathy, which is a condition very frequently encountered among athletes.

SHOULDER

Injuries to the rotator cuff are a very common source for dysfunction in athletes at all sports and levels of competition. Injuries to the rotator cuff can result from a direct blow, falling on an outstretched arm, or chronic overuse. Injuries are classified by severity, from rotator cuff contusions, tendinopathies, to tears. Rotator cuff disease has been shown to increase with age from 9.7% under the age of 20 to 62% over the age of 80[1] and is the most common cause of shoulder pain in the general population.[2] Rotator cuff injuries are also very common in sports that require overhead activities, and these athletes must be monitored carefully. For example, a study done on Major League Baseball pitchers showed that pitchers with rotator cuff injuries that needed surgery eventually had a decline in their performance leading up to surgical intervention.[3]

Biomechanics

The biomechanics of injury for the rotator cuff is thought to occur from repetitive activities with eccentric contraction particularly during the deceleration phase of throwing.[2] The articular side is more commonly torn than the bursal side of the rotator cuff and is often seen in these athletes.[4] The supraspinatus tendon is most often injured in a rotator cuff injury. This muscle is responsible for abduction and external rotation of the shoulder, but it is difficult to isolate during a physical examination due to the mechanics of the other rotator cuff muscles, which limits the accuracy of the clinical examination.[4]

Clinical Presentation

The clinical presentation of rotator cuff injuries may depend on the severity of injury. A thorough history of the shoulder injury should be taken into account, which should include a detailed mechanism of injury. Overhead athletes may present with a glenohumeral internal rotation deficit (GIRD), which is caused by muscular and capsular tightness.[5,6] These athletes will lose 20° or greater internal rotation in the dominant shoulder when at 90° of abduction.

Evaluation

Imaging should be done with plain radiographs to rule out bony injury, such as a Hill-Sachs deformity or a Bankart lesion of the glenoid. These lesions would lead a clinician to suspect rotator cuff injury or labral tear.[7] The bony defect itself does not require treatment; however, the associated glenohumeral instability is often coexistent with anterior labral injuries, which may require surgical repair. MRI scan is thought to be the gold standard to assess the integrity of the rotator cuff tendon and musculature, but musculoskeletal ultrasound also allows dynamic assessment.[8] Ultrasound has a very high sensitivity in diagnosing complete tendon tears but may be difficult to visualize the entire rotator cuff, which may make it difficult to identify partial rotator cuff tears.[9,10] The MRI allows better evaluation of the labrum and articular cartilage.

Management

Management of rotator cuff injuries is guided by the type of injury and severity and is initially treated either conservatively or surgically, based on the patient's age, size of and location of the tear, and activity limitations. A complete tear requires surgery. The initial therapy for rotator cuff tendinopathy typically consists of rest, ice, and nonsteroidal anti-inflammatory drugs (NSAIDs) and early rehabilitation with range of motion and eccentric exercises. In patients with GIRD and chronic tightness of the posterior rotator cuff or capsule, the modified sleeper stretch and the modified cross-body stretch are 2 common exercises that have been shown to be effective.[11]

In the elite athlete, there are many other factors for the treating clinician to consider. These considerations include sport, level of contact, positional demands, time of year, and both postseason and financial implications. It is imperative to identify these injuries, because they can also have a major impact on playing career and can limit their ability to participate in their sport. For example, in 1 study, it was shown that draft-eligible football players with an injury to the rotator cuff were significantly less likely to be drafted than those without a previous rotator cuff injury.[3]

ELBOW

Overuse injuries of the elbow and forearm are very common in athletes. Pain may come from within the joint or the surrounding soft tissue structures, such as the medial and lateral epicondyles. Sports that involve throwing or racquet sports, which use repetitive elbow flexion-extension or pronation-supination of the wrist, may cause stress injuries that lead to these syndromes. Tendinopathies about the elbow account for most of the pathologic condition in patients presenting with elbow pain and most commonly at the lateral epicondyle.[12]

Biomechanics

The elbow consists of 3 true joints that function as 1 joint: the humeroulnar joint, the humeroradial joint, and the proximal radioulnar joint.[13,14] The humeroulnar joint is a hinge joint and allows flexion and extension. The humeroradial joint also functions as a hinge joint, but also allows rotation of the radial head on the capitellum of the humerus. The radioulnar joint permits supination and pronation of the proximal elbow. The ligamentous structures are not true ligaments and function as thickenings of the capsules, which are divided into lateral and medial structures. The medial collateral ligament (MCL) provides valgus support of the elbow, whereas the lateral ulnar collateral ligament provides varus stability. The annular ligament maintains the radial head position in the radial notch of the humerus. Dynamic stability is provided by the muscle groups in the elbow: the biceps brachii, brachioradialis, and brachialis muscles. The triceps and anconeus muscles allow elbow extension, whereas the supinator and biceps brachii muscles provide supination. Pronation is achieved through the pronator quadratus, pronator teres, and flexor carpi radialis muscles.

Repetitive elbow flexion may cause biceps tendinopathy or anterior capsular strain. Activities that involve forceful elbow extension, such as throwing, can cause triceps tendinosis or posterior impingement syndrome. Activities that promote forced valgus stress on the elbow can also cause injuries to the lateral structures, such as the ulnar nerve, or olecranon stress fractures. The lateral epicondyle, which is most often affected according to observational studies, occurs with a frequency 7 to 10 times that of medial epicondylitis.[15] The reported incidence may approach 1% to 3% in the general population.[16,17] Most of these patients are in the age range of 30 to

40 years and develop lateral epicondylitis as a result of occupational overuse rather than sporting activities.[18,19]

Lateral epicondylitis is caused by repetitive stress affecting most frequently the extensor carpi radialis brevis (ECRB). The constant overload generates microtrauma in the tendons and muscles of the lateral epicondyle, which results in angiofibroblastic hyperplasia. Chronic epicondylitis, or rather epicondylosis, is more a degenerative process than an inflammatory process. As the tendon becomes repetitively injured, calcified tissues begin to form within the surrounding tissues, thus creating more diseased tendon. Tennis is the classic example of a sport in which this condition happens more frequently because of specific activities involved, and lateral epicondylitis is classically coined tennis elbow because of the prevalence of this condition in these athletes. Reports have estimated that almost half of all tennis players will present with lateral epicondylitis at some time during their sporting career.[20] The biomechanics of tennis are responsible, which require a certain grip and return shots that require wide-ranging use of forearm extensors. Incorrect technique is one of the factors that is most frequently cited to cause lateral epicondylitis.[21]

Clinical Presentation

A detailed history and mechanism of injury will determine the diagnosis. Popping, catching, clicking, and locking are mechanical symptoms that suggest an intraarticular pathologic condition, whereas instability symptoms suggest ligamentous injury just as in other joints. Different sports and occupations require stresses on the various structures of the elbow. An occupational history must be considered because many skilled or assembly line workers perform the same motions over and over that may put them at risk for overuse syndromes of the elbow just like athletes. In athletes with lateral epicondylitis, a specific account of the athlete's grip, swing, or throwing phase that reproduces symptoms should be asked about. Recent change in mechanics or equipment should be inquired about as well. Finally, the specific activity eliciting pain should be determined. For instance, pain during tennis may be exacerbated through backhand shots and also may radiate to the forearm, wrist, hand, and shoulder. As the tendinopathy worsens, simple activities of daily living, such as picking up items or turning a door handle, may become painful.

The physical examination should focus on the location of the pain using specific provocative maneuvers in order to obtain an accurate diagnosis.[13] The medial elbow should be evaluated for concomitant injury because there are athletes who have concomitant medial and lateral epicondylitis, also coined "country club elbow."[15] On the medial aspect of the elbow, the flexor-pronator mass originates from the medial epicondyle. Point tenderness over the medial epicondyle may represent epicondylitis, MCL injury, or fracture. The integrity of the MCL is most commonly tested with the valgus stress test or the milking maneuver. The lateral elbow should be examined by palpating of bony landmarks, the lateral collateral ligament, and the locating the "soft spot." The "soft spot" is the best location to detect an effusion in the elbow. The radiocapitellar joint is also palpated for tenderness with dynamic pronation and supination, which may be indicated with fracture or degenerative arthritis. For medial epicondylitis, the point of maximal tenderness is at the insertion of the flexor-pronator mass, 5 to 10 mm distal and anterior to the medial epicondyle. Pain with resisted pronation may be a very sensitive finding for medial epicondylitis but can also be elicited with resisted wrist flexion.[22] In lateral epicondylitis, maximal tenderness is typically about 1 cm distal to the epicondyle at the origin of the ECRB. These athletes may have decreased grip strength with resisted wrist supination and extension.[22]

Evaluation

Plain radiographs can be ordered initially in order to rule out medial or lateral epicondyle avulsions, loose bodies, or degenerative joint disease of the elbow particularly if the injury is acute.[23] Calcification of the common extensor or flexor tendon can be found in chronic cases of tendinosis. An olecranon stress fractures line or even loose bodies in the fossa can cause posterior impingement syndrome. MRI is preferred for chronic elbow pain because it can delineate soft tissue injuries and also show stress fractures or the bone edema at the fracture site. With MRI, the extent of tendon degeneration in a tendinosis can also be evaluated.[23] Musculoskeletal ultrasound requires a skilled clinician but allows for a dynamic evaluation of the elbow. Ultrasonography has a reported sensitivity of 64% to 82% for the diagnosis of medial and lateral elbow tendinopathy, compared with a sensitivity of 90% to 100% with MRI and is also less expensive.[24]

Management

Initial management of lateral epicondylitis is conservative treatment, such as activity modification, counterforce braces, NSAIDs, and physical therapy. Nonoperative management of lateral epicondylitis will result in successful resolution of symptoms in 90% of patients.[25] Studies on corticosteroid injections for these conditions found only short-term improvement but were equivocal at 1-year follow-up in the groups studied.[26,27] Platelet-rich plasma (PRP) injections have been shown to be effective in reducing pain and symptoms in the treatment of elbow epicondylosis.[28] Some studies have showed that PRP is superior to corticosteroid injections in pain relief, but there is mixed and limited evidence for long-term outcomes.[29] Failure to improve after 6 to 12 months of conservative management would lead to a consideration for surgical intervention.

Proper equipment may be helpful in preventing this injury, such as the size of the racquet grip, and the string tension of the racquet should also be individualized. For nonelite tennis players who can tolerate decreased performance, a wide profile can be recommended because of its larger area of minimum vibration ("sweet spot") when making a shot.

WRIST

Wrist pain often can be a challenging presenting injury to patients and athletes. It can be classified as acute pain caused by a trauma or as subacute/chronic pain. Acute wrist pain can be caused by conditions such as contusions, fractures, ligament sprains, and instability. Chronic pain usually results from overuse or may be caused by previous injury. Patients with these injuries may have a history of repetitive wrist movement, either occupationally or recreationally.

Determining the cause of ulnar-sided wrist pain in particular may be difficult, mainly because of the complex anatomic and biomechanical properties of that side of the wrist.

Biomechanics

The wrist biomechanics functions as a joint that connects the forearm and the hand. It is made up from the distal radius, the ulna, the carpal bones, and the bases of the metacarpals. The mobility of the wrist is determined by these structures and the attachments of the various ligaments. The wrist joint consists of the distal radioulnar joint (DRUJ), which is the articulation of the distal radius and ulnar head. It functions in both pronation and supination of the wrist as the radius shortens in pronation and lengthens during supination in relation to the ulna. The triangular fibrocartilage complex (TFCC) on the ulnar side of the wrist serves as a cushion for the ulnar carpus and helps stabilize the DRUJ. The 8 bones of the carpus also function as a link between the distal radius and ulna and the metacarpals of the hand to assist with both flexion and extension of the hand, and ulnar and radial deviation of the wrist.

Clinical Presentation

A detailed history alone may lead to a specific diagnosis in approximately 70% of patients who have wrist pain.[30] A history should be obtained to ascertain if the wrist pain was caused by an acute injury or by repetitive motions of the wrist. Mechanical symptoms, such as grinding, snaps, clicks, or clunks, each may have a unique pathologic condition. A click usually may indicate 2 bones rubbing against each other, as in triquetral instability. A snap is often associated with a subluxing tendon. Clunks may indicate joint subluxation, such as midcarpal instability. Special provocative tests (eg, triquetrolunate ballottement, ulnar ballottement, midcarpal shifting) can be performed to confirm the suspected pathologic condition.

The wrist can be divided into areas to focus on owing to their interrelated to structures: dorsal radial, dorsal central, dorsal ulnar, volar ulnar, volar central, and volar radial sections. The dorsal ulnar zone is important because of injury to the DRUJ or TFCC.

The DRUJ should be evaluated by palpating over the distal radius and lunate articulation and distal ulna. Pain that occurs with pronation and supination of the wrist may suggest injury to the DRUJ. The examiner must be careful to rotate the forearm at the wrist, not at the hand. Squeezing the ulna and radius together causes pain, crepitation, or a snap in a patient with DRUJ disease. The TFCC is palpated just distal to the ulna and may indicate tears to the TFCC.

The TFCC load test may reveal these tears by applying an axial load while the patient is ulnar deviating the affected wrist. In addition, forearm pronation and supination are usually pain free with TFCC tears.

The piano-key test involves depressing the distal ulna from dorsal to volar with the hand pronated. A positive result is characterized by painful laxity in the affected wrist compared with the contralateral wrist. The results are usually positive in cases of DRUJ synovitis.

A positive ulnar compression test may indicate possible degeneration or inflammation. To perform this test, compress the ulnar head against the sigmoid notch. A positive result is exacerbation of pain, which suggests arthritis or instability. In addition, with ulnar compression, dorsal or volar subluxation may be noted.

Evaluation

Imaging should include plain radiographs with posteroanterior (PA) and lateral views of the wrist. Musculoskeletal ultrasound has been shown to be a useful modality in the evaluation of wrist injuries particularly for ligamentous structures and the TFCC.[22] This imaging modality has been particularly useful in evaluating ganglion cysts, tendons, and tendon sheaths. When the diagnosis remains unclear, MRI is the preferred examination. However, if a TFCC tear is suspected, arthrography should be used to confirm the diagnosis.[31]

Management

Tears to the TFCC can be caused by acute trauma or from chronic degenerative causes. Degenerative lesions are the result of repetitive injuries that involve loading on the ulnar wrist, but many of these lesions are asymptomatic and therefore treated conservatively. Traumatic lesions without pain or instability are also treated conservatively. Conservative treatment may include a long arm cast for 6 weeks, NSAIDs, or corticosteroid injections. If the TFCC tear has associated instability or if injuries fail to respond to conservative management, those injuries should be referred to a hand surgeon for TFCC debridement and ulnar shortening.[32]

HAND

The fingers are the part of the upper extremity used for touch, feel, and fine-motor skills and to perform activities of daily living. Finger and metacarpal fractures are reportedly the most common sports-related fractures commonly seen in the office.[33,34] Most of the injuries to the fingers, if seen, diagnosed, and managed appropriately, do not threaten limb viability, long-term function, or return to play. Finger injuries are most important to catch and diagnose accurately because the greatest morbidity from these injuries are from delay in diagnosis or missed injuries, leading to deformity and loss of function.

Biomechanics

The second through fifth fingers all have proximal, middle, and distal phalanges with 3 hinged joints: distal interphalangeal (DIP), proximal interphalangeal (PIP), and metacarpal phalangeal (MCP). The thumb only has a distal and proximal phalanx and an interphalangeal (IP) and MCP joint. The volar plates, which are collateral ligaments for the fingers, provide joint stability.[35]

The extensor tendons of the fingers divide into a central slip, which extends the PIP and then splits into 2 lateral bands, which extend the DIP. This anatomy is important in the development of central slip avulsions or boutonniere deformities. Central slip extensor tendon injury is caused when the PIP is forcibly flexed while actively extended. Volar dislocation of the PIP joint also can cause central slip ruptures. The flexor tendons include the flexor digitorum superficialis and the flexor digitorum profundus (FDP). The flexor digitorum superficialis tendon attaches to the base of the middle phalanx and flexes the PIP joint. The FDP tendon is located under and splits the flexor digitorum superficialis tendon. It attaches to the base of the distal phalanx and flexes the DIP. Disruption of the FDP tendon can occur when an athlete's finger gets caught in another player's jersey, therefore described as jersey finger. The mechanism of injury is from forced, passive extension of the DIP joint during active flexion of DIP.

Clinical Presentation

Jersey finger is caused by a traumatic avulsion of FDP from the distal phalanx.

There may be an avulsed palmar fragment from distal phalanx; the ring finger is affected most commonly and is often missed for several weeks. The diagnosis is based on the mechanism of injury and inability to flex the DIP joint. On physical examination, a tendon stump may be palpated in the palm or along the digit; bony avulsions can be trapped at flexor sheath (A4 pulley over middle phalanx). However, soft tissue swelling can lead to false physical examination findings, and the point of maximal tenderness is not sufficient at identifying the avulsed tendon stump.

A rupture of the central extensor tendon of the finger occurs at the PIP joint. The mechanism of injury and inability to completely extend the injured finger at the PIP joint indicate this type of injury. Plain radiographs may not show the avulsed fragment in these injuries and may only show the flexion of the PIP joint. Surgical repair of the rupture should be scheduled without delay.[36] Most injuries at this joint occur from forced extension, not flexion, and result in a volar plate rupture.[36] If swelling and pain make evaluation the of an acute dislocation injury difficult, splinting in the "safe hand" position for 72 hours while icing the injured finger will make it possible to do a more detailed follow-up examination. Extended periods of splinting can make the PIP joint stiff and more difficult to treat than the original injury.[37,38] If the rupture of the central extensor tendon is undetected or not treated, a Boutonniere deformity, in which the PIP joint is flexed and the DIP joint is hyperextended, may be the likely result.[36]

Evaluation

Plain radiographs (PA, lateral, oblique) are done first to identify if an avulsed fragment is present. Ultrasound is one of the best ways to differentiate between partial and full-thickness rupture and localizing the distal tendon stump.[36] MRI is reserved for precise evaluation of the tendon edges, which may aid the surgeon in operative planning.

Management

Management of jersey finger involves splinting with the DIP and PIP in slight flexion. More commonly, the tendon will be retracted to PIP. Referral may be delayed a few weeks, but caution should be taken because the tendon may still retract further. Jersey finger needs surgical reattachment of the flexor tendon within 7 to 10 days. If the tendon is retracted to the palm, scarring may be irreversible because there is no blood supply. Athletes typically return to play in 12 weeks with protected activity, then full gripping/grasping can be allowed. If open reduction internal fixation is performed, then 4 to 6 weeks of protected activity is advised. All of these cases need physical/occupational therapy when healed.

In patients with PIP joint injuries, the PIP joint should be thought of as a hinge joint that is kept in alignment by a soft tissue "envelope" that consists of the joint capsule, the volar plate, collateral ligaments, and the central slip.[39] If a dislocation occurs, at least 2 of these structures are injured. Evaluation of an acutely injured finger may be difficult, and splinting the patient in the "safe hand" position for 72 hours while icing frequently allows a more detailed follow-up examination. Careful palpation allows one to ascertain which structures are injured and the type of splinting to be used. Placing the patient in a dorsal splint that allows flexion of the DIP and MP joints while the PIP is splinted in extension is a nonsurgical way to treat an incomplete central slip injury. Patients unable to extend their PIP joint require prompt surgical consult.

SUMMARY

Upper-extremity injuries in athletes are common conditions that must be immediately identified by the clinician in order to return the athlete to play and normal function. When the understanding of normal physioanatomy and biomechanics for each joint is partnered with a thorough history and an evidence-based physical examination, an accurate diagnosis and treatment plan can be made. Point-of-care musculoskeletal ultrasound for these conditions is proven to be helpful and inexpensive. Prompt recognition of urgent conditions that require orthopedic referral is also vital, but if recognized immediately, can provide the athlete the optimal outcome.

DISCLOSURE

The author has nothing to disclose.

REFERENCES

1. Teunis T, Lubberts B, Reilly BT, et al. A systematic review and pooled analysis of the prevalence of rotator cuff disease with increasing age. J Shoulder Elbow Surg 2014;23(12):1913–21.
2. van der Windt DA, Koes BW, de Jong BA, et al. Shoulder disorders in general practice: incidence, patient characteristics, and management. Ann Rheum Dis 1995;54(12):959–64.
3. Namdari S, Baldwin K, Ahn A, et al. Performance after rotator cuff tear and operative treatment: a case-control study of Major League Baseball pitchers. J Athl Train 2011;46(3):296–302.
4. Dela Rosa TL, Wang AW, Zheng MH. Tendinosis of the rotator cuff: a review. J Musculoskel Res 2001;5:143.
5. Burkhart SS, Morgan CD, Kibler WB. The disabled throwing shoulder: spectrum of pathology Part III: the SICK scapula, scapular dyskinesis, the kinetic chain, and rehabilitation. Arthroscopy 2003;19(6):641–61.
6. Carvalho CD, Cohen C, Belangero PS, et al. Partial rotator cuff injury in athletes: bursal or articular? Rev Bras Ortop 2015;50(4):416–21.
7. Widjaja AB, Tran A, Bailey M, et al. Correlation between Bankart and Hill-Sachs lesions in anterior shoulder dislocation. ANZ J Surg 2006;76(6):436–8.
8. Lew HL, Chen CP, Wang TG, et al. Introduction to musculoskeletal diagnostic ultrasound: examination of the upper limb. Am J Phys Med Rehabil 2007;86(4): 310–21.
9. Rutten MJ, Jager GJ, Kiemeney LA. Ultrasound detection of rotator cuff tears: observer agreement related to increasing experience. AJR Am J Roentgenol 2010;195(6):W440–6.
10. Schipper ON, Dunn JH, Ochiai DH, et al. Nirschl surgical technique for concomitant lateral and medial elbow tendinosis: a retrospective review of 53 elbows with a mean follow-up of 11.7 years. Am J Sports Med 2011;39(5):972–6.
11. Weiss LJ, Wang D, Hendel M, et al. Management of rotator cuff injuries in the elite athlete. Curr Rev Musculoskelet Med 2018;11(1):102–12.
12. Laratta J, Caldwell JM, Lombardi J, et al. Evaluation of common elbow pathologies: a focus on physical examination. Phys Sportsmed 2017;45(2):184–90.
13. Budoff JE, Nirschl RP. Elbow complaints: keys to effective examination. Consultant 2001;2:509–16.
14. Burkhart SS, Morgan CD, Kibler WB. The disabled throwing shoulder: spectrum of pathology Part I: pathoanatomy and biomechanics. Arthroscopy 2003;19(4): 404–20.
15. Ciccotti MC, Schwartz MA, Ciccotti MG. Diagnosis and treatment of medial epicondylitis of the elbow. Clin Sports Med 2004;23(4):693–705, xi.
16. Struijs PA, Kerkhoffs GM, Assendelft WJ, et al. Conservative treatment of lateral epicondylitis: brace versus physical therapy or a combination of both–a randomized clinical trial. Am J Sports Med 2004;32(2):462–9.
17. Taljanovic MS, Sheppard JE, Jones MD, et al. Sonography and sonoarthrography of the scapholunate and lunotriquetral ligaments and triangular fibrocartilage disk: initial experience and correlation with arthrography and magnetic resonance arthrography. J Ultrasound Med 2008;27(2):179–91.
18. Garg R, Adamson GJ, Dawson PA, et al. A prospective randomized study comparing a forearm strap brace versus a wrist splint for the treatment of lateral epicondylitis. J Shoulder Elbow Surg 2010;19(4):508–12.

19. Gibbs DB, Lynch TS, Gombera MM, et al. Preexisting rotator cuff tears as a predictor of outcomes in National Football League athletes. Sports Health 2016;8(3): 250–4.
20. Silva R, Santos MB. Tennis elbow: a survey among 839 tennis players with and without injury. Med Sci Tennis. 2008;13(1):36–41.
21. Roetert EP, Brody H, Dillman CJ, et al. The biomechanics of tennis elbow. An integrated approach. Clin Sports Med 1995;14(1):47–57.
22. Van Hofwegen C, Baker CL. Epicondylitis in the athlete's elbow. Clin Sports Med 2010;29(4):577–97.
23. Stevens KJ, McNally EG. Magnetic resonance imaging of the elbow in athletes. Clin Sports Med 2010;29(4):521–53.
24. Walz DM, Newman JS, Konin GP, et al. Epicondylitis: pathogenesis, imaging, and treatment. Radiographics 2010;30(1):167–84.
25. Coonrad RW, Hooper WR. Tennis elbow: its course, natural history, conservative and surgical management. J Bone Joint Surg Am 1973;55(6):1177–82.
26. Hay EM, Paterson SM, Lewis M, et al. Pragmatic randomised controlled trial of local corticosteroid injection and naproxen for treatment of lateral epicondylitis of elbow in primary care. BMJ 1999;319(7215):964–8.
27. Kane SF, Lynch JH, Taylor JC. Evaluation of elbow pain in adults. Am Fam Physician 2014;89(8):649–57.
28. Taylor SA, Hannafin JA. Evaluation and management of elbow tendinopathy. Sports Health 2012;4(5):384–93.
29. Kwapisz A, Prabhakar S, Compagnoni R, et al. Platelet-rich plasma for elbow pathologies: a descriptive review of current literature. Curr Rev Musculoskelet Med 2018;11(4):598–606.
30. Forman TA, Forman SK, Rose NE. A clinical approach to diagnosing wrist pain. Am Fam Physician 2005;72(9):1753–8.
31. Albastaki U, Sophocleous D, Göthlin J, et al. Magnetic resonance imaging of the triangular fibrocartilage complex lesions: a comprehensive clinicoradiologic approach and review of the literature. J Manipulative Physiol Ther 2007;30(7): 522–6.
32. Yao J, Dantuluri P, Osterman AL. A novel technique of all-inside arthroscopic triangular fibrocartilage complex repair. Arthroscopy 2007;23(12):1357.e1-4.
33. Court-Brown CM, Wood AM, Aitken S. The epidemiology of acute sports-related fractures in adults. Injury 2008;39(12):1365–72.
34. da Silva RT. Sports injuries of the upper limbs. Rev Bras Ortop 2010;45(2): 122–31.
35. Freiberg A. Management of proximal interphalangeal joint injuries. Can J Plast Surg 2007;15(4):199–203.
36. Daniels JM, Zook EG, Lynch JM. Hand and wrist injuries: Part II. Emergent evaluation. Am Fam Physician 2004;69(8):1949–56.
37. Oetgen ME, Dodds SD. Non-operative treatment of common finger injuries. Curr Rev Musculoskelet Med 2008;1(2):97–102.
38. Perron AD, Brady WJ, Keats TE, et al. Orthopedic pitfalls in the emergency department: closed tendon injuries of the hand. Am J Emerg Med 2001;19(1): 76–80.
39. Freiberg A, Pollard BA, Macdonald MR, et al. Management of proximal interphalangeal joint injuries. Hand Clin 2006;22(3):235–42.

Hip and Knee Injuries

Stephen M. Carek, MD, CAQSM

KEYWORDS

• Hip injuries • Knee injuries • Osteoarthritis • Sports injuries

KEY POINTS

- Hip and knee injuries are a common presentation to primary care offices and encompass a wide spectrum of injuries, from acute trauma to chronic degenerative conditions.
- Understanding clinical clues, components of the history, physical examination, and appropriate imaging studies can guide a primary care provider toward a correct diagnosis and treatment plan.
- Most musculoskeletal injuries that present can initially be treated with rest, ice, anti-inflammatories, activity modification, and consideration of physical therapy to correct underlying muscle weakness or biomechanical deficiencies.

INTRODUCTION

Hip and knee injuries commonly present to primary care providers and represent a broad differential, presenting a diagnostic challenge. It is important to understand the anatomy of each joint because it can provide helpful clues in determining the etiology of a patient's pain as well as appropriate interventions for treatment. Knee pain accounts for approximately one-third of musculoskeletal problems seen in primary care settings and is prevalent in physically active patients, with up to 54% of athletes having some degree of knee pain each year. Hip pain accounts for up to 9% of high school athletes[1] and up to 14% of adults 60 years and older who report significant hip pain on most days.[2] Collectively, these injuries can be a source of disability, restricting the ability to compete, work, or perform activities of daily living.

HIP INJURIES
Anatomy

The hip is a ball-and-socket synovial joint designed to allow multiaxial motion while transferring loads between the upper and lower body. The acetabular rim is lined with fibrocartilage, the labrum, which provides depth and stability to the joint. The articular joint is lined with hyaline cartilage that dissipates shear and compressive forces during load bearing and hip motion. The wide range of motion provided by the hip joint is enabled by the bony morphology, joint capsule, and ligaments, as

Department of Family Medicine, University of South Carolina, School of Medicine–Greenville, Center for Family Medicine - Greenville, 877 West Faris Road, Greenville, SC 29605, USA.
E-mail address: Stephen.carek@prismahealth.org

Prim Care Clin Office Pract 47 (2020) 115–131
https://doi.org/10.1016/j.pop.2019.10.006
0095-4543/20/© 2019 Elsevier Inc. All rights reserved.

primarycare.theclinics.com

well as the complex system of interplaying muscle groups surrounding it. The flexor muscles include the iliopsoas, rectus femoris, pectineus, and sartorius muscles. Hip extension is provided by the gluteus maximus and hamstring muscle groups (biceps femoris, semitendinosis, and semimembranosus). Muscles inserting around the greater trochanter, the gluteus medius and minimus, piriformis, obturator externus and internus, and quadratus femoris, allow for abduction, adductions, and internal and external rotation.

Evaluation of Hip Pain

History

Several components of the patient's history can help to narrow the differential diagnosis of hip pain. In prepubescent and adolescent patients, congenital malformations of the femoroacetabular joint, avulsion fractures, or apophyseal or epiphyseal injuries should be considered. In skeletally mature individuals, hip pain is often a result of musculotendinous strain or ligamentous sprain, contusion, or bursitis. In older adults, degenerative osteoarthritis and fractures should be considered first. Inquire about recent trauma or inciting activity, factors that increase or decrease pain, mechanism of injury, and time of onset. An important component of a patient's description of hip pain is the location, which is typically localized to 1 of 3 basic anatomic regions: the anterior hip and groin, posterior hip and buttock, and lateral hip.

Physical examination

The hip examination should evaluate the hip, back, abdomen, and vascular and neurologic systems. It should start with a gait analysis and stance assessment, followed by evaluation of the patient in seated supine, lateral, and prone positions. Additional physical examination tests for the evaluation of hip pain are summarized in **Table 1**.

Imaging

Radiographs Radiography of the hip should be performed if there is any concern for fracture, dislocation, or stress injury. Imaging should include an anteroposterior view of the pelvis and frog-leg lateral view of the symptomatic hip.[3]

Magnetic resonance imaging Magnetic resonance imaging (MRI) is the preferred imaging modality if plain radiography does not identify specific pathology to explain a patient's symptoms.[4] An MR arthrogram of the hip should be considered if a labral tear is suspected, because it increases sensitivity from 66% to 87%.[5,6]

Common Hip Injuries

Osteoarthritis

Osteoarthritis of the hip is characterized by the loss of articular cartilage within the hip joint. It is the most likely diagnosis in older adults with decreased range of motion and a gradual onset of symptoms. Pain is typically described as a constant, deep, and ache that is worsened with prolonged periods of standing and weight bearing. On examination, the patient typically presents with a decreased range of motion and pain elicited on the extremes of motion. Plain radiographs demonstrate the presence of asymmetrical joint space narrowing, osteophyte formation, subchondral sclerosis, and cyst formation.

The initial treatment is often nonsurgical and consists of pain control with acetaminophen or nonsteroidal anti-inflammatory drugs, activity modification, and use of assistive devices for protective weight bearing.[7–9] In obese patients, weight loss should be emphasized in addition to conservative measures. Non–weight-bearing exercise and hip strengthening are occasionally helpful, but run the risk of exacerbating symptoms.

Table 1
Special examination maneuvers for the hip

Test	Description	Positive Finding	Conditions Associated with Positive Finding
Trendelenburg test	Observe the patient standing on 1 leg.	The pelvis drops below the level on the side the patient is not standing on.	Greater trochanteric pain syndrome Gluteus medius weakness
FABER test	With the patient supine, place the affected hip in flexion, abduction and external rotation while the patient's foot is on the other knee (figure-of-4). Stabilize the pelvis with your hand on the contralateral anterior superior iliac spine and press down on the thigh of the affected side.	Posterior pain localized to the sacroiliac joint, lumbar spine or posterior hip; groin pain with the test is sensitive for intra-articular pathology	Hip labral tear, femoral acetabular impingement, osteoarthritis, sacroiliac joint dysfunction, iliopsoas bursitis
FADIR test	With the patient supine, raise the affected hip and knee in 90° of flexion. Supporting the knee and ankle, then the adducts over the midline and internally rotates the hip.	Anterior or anterolateral hip pain	Hip labral tear, loose bodies, chondral lesions, femoral acetabular impingement
Log roll test	With the patient supine, internally and externally rotate the relaxed lower extremity.	Pain in the anterior hip or groin, particularly with internal rotation	Hip osteoarthritis, femoral head osteonecrosis, slipped capital femoral epiphysis
Ober test	With the patient lying in a lateral position with the affect side up and stabilizing the hip, support the knee and flex it to 90°. Then extend and abduct the hip while releasing the knee support and sliding the hand toward the bottom of the leg. Observe the knee and thigh lowering toward the table.	The patient's knee is unable to adduct the leg parallel to the table in a neutral position.	Iliotibial band syndrome, external snapping hip, greater trochanteric pain syndrome

(continued on next page)

Table 1 (continued)			
Test	Description	Positive Finding	Conditions Associated with Positive Finding
Thomas test	Have the patient sit at the end of the examination table with the legs over the edge of the table far enough that the table edge will not contact the posterior aspect of the calves. The patient then assumes a supine position with the legs hanging off the end of the table and pulls one hip into maximum flexion.	—	Greater trochanteric pain

Abbreviation: FADIR, Flexion, Adduction, and Internal Rotation.

Intra-articular injections, either guided with ultrasound imaging or fluoroscopy, are helpful for acute exacerbation of symptoms if conservative measures fail.[10] If nonsurgical treatment fails, most are treated with total hip arthroplasty.

Femoroacetabular impingement
Typically seen in young and active patients, femoroacetabular impingement is typically described as an insidious onset of pain that is worsened with sitting, rising from a seat, kicking, or extreme motion of the hip. This condition occurs due to osseous deformities on the acetabular rim, the femoral head-neck junction, or both that abut at extremes of hip motion and cause injury to the acetabular labrum and cartilage.[11] Patients can range from teenagers to middle ages. Pain tends to be in the anterior groin with occasional radiation to the lateral hip or anterior thigh. Associated catching, locking, or clicking also may be present. The physical examination reveals decreased hip flexion and internal rotation compared with the opposite extremity and classically is associated with a positive Flexion, Adduction, and Internal Rotation maneuver (see **Table 1**), also known as the impingement sign.[12] Anteroposterior and lateral radiographs of the hip are indicated for patients with pain and limited internal rotation of the hip. The classic radiographic features are a loss of femoral head-neck offset, also referred to as a cam deformity, or a prominent anterior acetabular rim, also referred to as a pincer abnormality.[13,14] MR arthrography is the hip is the most accurate modality for demonstrating associated labral ears and osseous abnormalities.[4]

The initial treatment is typically nonsurgical and consists of pain control, activity modification, and physical therapy focusing on hip range of motion and strengthening. However, this literature is limited and no consensus has determined specific therapies or duration of therapy that would confer a benefit for patient.[15] Intra-articular hip injections with a combination of a local anesthetic and a corticosteroids have a limited therapeutic benefit, but are also a diagnostic tool if the etiology of a patient's pain is unclear.[16] If refractory to nonoperative treatment, surgery may be indicated. Although short-term improvements in pain and function are documented,[17] long-term benefit over improvement in pain or function compared with nonsurgical interventions is limited.[18]

Acetabular labral tear

Acetabular labral tears usually have an insidious onset, but occasionally begin after a traumatic event or injury. Most tears are thought to be a product of repetitive micro-trauma through repetitive pivoting on a loaded femur.[19] The presence of a cam-type femoroacetabular impingement or developmental dysplasia of the hip can increase risk of labral tears.[20] They are typically a dull or sharp groin pain with pain that radiates to the anterior thigh, lateral hip, and buttock. Mechanical symptoms, such as catching or painful clicking with activity, are also present at times.[21] MR arthrography is considered the diagnostic test of choice.[4]

Conservative management with physical therapy directed to unloading the damaged labrum and improving hip joint neuromotor control helps to manage symptoms and improve function of the hip.[22] Should conservative measures fail, hip arthroscopy and labral repair and correction of underlying osseous pathomorphology may be pursued. Labral repair has shown to improve patient's reported pain and function, decrease time to return to sport, and can potentially decrease the risk of long-term osteoarthritis.[23,24]

Snapping hip syndrome (coxa saltans)

Snapping hip is characterized by an audible snapping, often accompanied by pain, which usually occurs with the flexion and extension of the hip during exercise or daily activities. There are 3 types of snapping hip: the slipping of the iliotibial (IT) band over the greater trochanter, sliding of the iliopsoas tendon over the pectineal eminence of the pelvis, or owing to intra-articular tears of the acetabular labrum or lose bodies.[25] Physical examination can demonstrate either a palpable or audible snapping when the hip extends from a flexed position, or having the patient rotate the hip while holding it in an adducted position. Although snapping hip is usually a clinical diagnosis, plain radiographs can be helpful in evaluating for bony pathology or intra-articular hip disease. MR arthrography can help to rule out a labral tear of the acetabulum. Dynamic ultrasound examination is useful in evaluating the various forms of snapping hip.[26]

If treatment is needed, exercises to stretch and strengthen the IT band, hip abductors, hip adductors, and hip flexors are recommended. A short course of nonsteroidal anti-inflammatories or injection of steroids into the iliopsoas bursa can decrease the discomfort associated with tendon snapping or resulting bursitis.[26,27] Recalcitrant cases are treated with surgery to lengthen the iliopsoas or IT band or correct intra-articular pathology attributed to the patient's symptoms.[28]

Stress fracture of the femoral neck

Hip pain exacerbated by repetitive weight bearing exercise and worsens with activity is concerning for development of a stress fracture. These injuries are considered high risk for transition to occult fracture if diagnosis is delayed.[29] MRI of the hip should be evaluated if no evidence for stress fracture or stress reaction is seen on plain radiographs.[30] Patients usually present with vague pain in the groin, anterior thigh, or knee that is associated with activity or weight bearing and usually subsides after cessation of activity.[31] Athletes or military recruits typically report an increase in exercise intensity or activity level in the few weeks preceding symptoms.

Stress fractures of the femoral neck are classified as tension side (lateral) or compression side (medial).[32] All tension-side stress fractures are treated surgically with internal fixation owing to their high tendency to displace. Compression-side stress fractures are treated with a period of non–weight-bearing and cessation of activity for 6 to 8 weeks. Surgery may be considered for those who demonstrate fracture progression or persistent symptoms despite appropriate nonsurgical treatment.[33]

Greater trochanteric pain syndrome

Lateral hip pain is most commonly referred to as greater trochanteric pain syndrome. Several disorders can lead to this type of pain, including IT band thickening, bursitis, and tears of the gluteus medius and minimus muscle attachment.[34] Pain is typically an atraumatic, insidious onset of symptoms from repetitive use and patients may endorse difficulty sleeping on the affected side as well as significant disability and reduction in quality of life.[35] Physical examination typically reveals tenderness over the lateral greater trochanter and exacerbated with active hip abduction.[36] Having the patient stand for 30 seconds on the affected leg is another physical examination technique with a high correlation to greater trochanteric pain syndrome.[37] Plain radiographs of the hip and pelvis are helpful to rule out bony abnormalities and intra-articular hip pathology, but are often unremarkable with isolated greater trochanteric pain syndrome.

Treatment consists of nonsteroidal anti-inflammatories, IT band stretching, activity modification, and a physical therapy regimen incorporating hip abduction strengthening.[38] Corticosteroid injections can be helpful in relieving pain and improving function as well when applied to a multimodal conservative plan.[39]

KNEE INJURIES
Anatomy

The knee is the largest joint in the body and a common source of athletics-related injuries. It is classified as a pivotal hinge joint, which allows for flexion and extension as well as a degree of internal and external rotation. The knee joint contains 4 bones—the femur, tibia, patella, and fibula—and consists of 3 articulating compartments—the medial tibiofemoral, lateral tibiofemoral, and patellofemoral—all of which share a synovial cavity. Articular cartilage within the joint allows for motion with minimal friction. The medial and lateral meniscus are fibrocartilage elements that act to cushion and decrease the effect of impact between the femur and tibia. Four ligaments aid in maintaining flexibility, stability and strength of the knee: the anterior cruciate ligament (ACL), the posterior cruciate ligament (PCL), the lateral collateral ligament, and the medial collateral ligament (MCL). The ACL and PCL function to prevent anterior and posterior translocation of the tibia relative to the femur, respectively. The MCL and lateral collateral ligament function to stabilize the knee from valgus and varus forces, respectively. Other structures that contribute to knee stability include the IT band and parts of the posterolateral corner. The extensor mechanism of the knee consists of the quadriceps muscles, the quadriceps tendon, and the patellar tendon. The hamstring muscles—the semitendinosus, semimembranosus, and the biceps femoris—are the primary flexors of the knee.

Evaluation of Knee Pain

History

Having the patient describe the knee pain is helpful when formulating a differential diagnosis. Clarification of pain quality, onset, location (anterior, posterior, medial, lateral), duration, and severity is essential to directing the workup of patient with knee pain. Common diagnostic categories for understanding the etiology of a patient's knee pain can be placed into 3 groups: acute pain after recent trauma or overuse, chronic knee pain associated with overuse, or knee pain without trauma or overuse, possibly associated with systemic signs or symptoms. It is also important to inquire about previous injuries, surgeries, any medications, systemic disease, or the presence of constitutional symptoms the patient may have. If the knee pain is caused by an acute injury, an understanding of the patient's ability to bear weight and any sensation of instability is important when determining what type of imaging or if surgical evaluation is required. Mechanical symptoms include locking, popping, or giving way of the knee. The presence of a knee effusion is likely indicative of an intra-articular injury, such as an ACL tear. An effusion that develops within a few hours of injury typically indicates a hemarthrosis, which commonly develops after rupture of the ACL or fracture of bone within the joint capsule. An effusion that develops more slowly or 1 to 2 days after injury is more likely to be a traumatic synovitis secondary to a meniscal or chondral pathology.

Physical examination

When evaluating a knee, it is important to perform the examination in a systematic manner to avoid missing findings that may assist in diagnosis. Perform the essential elements of the examination, such as inspection, palpation, and tests of motion and strength, in the same order and manner each time. Observing a patient's gait, alignment (valgus or varus), presence of swelling or joint effusion, muscle atrophy, or overlying skin changes is important as well. Normal limits of knee range of motion include extension from 0 to $-10°$ and flexion to 135°. Assessing for lateral patellar tracking (J sign) versus normal patellofemoral tracking during the range of motion examination. Neurovascular assessment, including sensation, deep tendon reflexes at the patella and Achilles, and palpation of the popliteal, dorsalis pedis, and posterior tibial pulses, should also be a part of a regular examination of the knee. Special tests, described in **Table 2**, are used to assess specific structures in the knee. These tests have varying accuracy and may be limited given extent of injury or presence of effusion.

Imaging

Radiographs The use of plain radiographs for knees in the outpatient primary care setting is typically reserved for chronic knee pain of more than 6 weeks duration or in the setting of an acute injury. The American College of Radiology Appropriateness criteria cite the Ottawa Knee Rule as a validated tool to determine if a patient requires a radiograph of the knee in the setting of an acute injury.[40] The Ottawa Knee rules indicate that any patient 55 years or older, an inability to bear weight for 4 steps immediately after injury or in the emergency department setting, an inability to flex the knee to 90°, or tenderness over the head of the fibula or isolated to the patella without other bony tenderness, as meeting criteria for knee radiographs.[41] The 3 recommended radiographic views are anteroposterior view, lateral view, and sunrise view (Merchant's view). If osteoarthritis is suspected, weight-bearing radiographs should be obtained to assess for joint space narrowing, subchondral sclerosis, osteophytes, and bony cysts.

Magnetic resonance imaging MRI is typically reserved for potential surgical indications such as a dislocation, an ACL or PCL tear, if fracture is suspected but absent on plain radiographs, a meniscal tear, vascular injury, loose body, or osteomyelitis.[42] MRI is useful if mechanical symptoms, such as painful clicking, locking, an inability to achieve full range of motion, or recurrent swelling or persistent pain, exist after a trial of conservative management.

Common Knee Injuries

Knee osteoarthritis

Knee osteoarthritis is typically encountered in patient older than 60 years or those with a previous knee injury or surgery. It can involve each of the 3 compartments of the knee, individually or in combination. Pain is typically aggravated by weight-bearing

Table 2
Special examination maneuvers for the knee

Test	Description	Positive Finding	Conditions Associated with Positive Finding
Anterior drawer test	Place the patient in a supine position with the hip flexed to 45° and the knee to 90°. Sit on the dorsum of the foot and wrap hand around the proximal tibia, placing the thumbs over the anteromedial and anterolateral joint lines. Push and pull the proximal leg, noting the degree of anterior translocation of the tibia relative to the femur, and feel for an endpoint where the ACL catches.	Translocation of the tibia no more than 6–8 mm or loss of a clear end-point	ACL tear
Lachman test	With the patient supine and the leg slightly externally rotated and flexed to 20–30°, stabilize the femur with one hand and use the other hand to apply posterior pressure and translocate the proximal tibia anteriorly relative to the distal femur	6–8 mm of translocation or loss of endpoint	ACL tear
Thessaly test	With the patient standing on the affected limb, load the meniscus with the knee flexed to 20° while internally and externally rotating the knee	Pain or catching sensation	Meniscal tear

(continued on next page)

Test	Description	Positive Finding	Conditions Associated with Positive Finding
Table 2 **(continued)**			
McMurray test	With the patient in a supine position, grasp the patients heel with 1 hand and place fingers and thumb of the other hand along the joint line of the knee. Passively flex the knee as much as possible and internally rotate the tibia, then extend the knee while maintaining internal rotation. Repeat full passive flexion and extension several times, then perform the same maneuver with the knee in external rotation.	Pain or mechanical clicking	Meniscal tear
Noble compression test	With the patient in the lateral decubitus position and the examiner standing behind them, the clinician places their thumb on the distal IT band just proximal to the lateral femoral epicondyle. Using the other hand, the examiner holds the patient's lower shin and flexes the knee from 0 to 60°.	Reproduced pain or clicking.	IT band syndrome

activities and alleviated with rest, but may experience morning stiffness that dissipates somewhat with activity. Common symptoms also include buckling or giving way, which is caused by reflex quadriceps inhibition or laxity from joint erosion. Findings on physical examination include decreased range of motion, crepitus, and mild joint effusion or synovial hypertrophy with palpable osteophytic changes at the knee joint. If osteoarthritis is suspected, weight-bearing radiographs of the knee can help to determine joint space narrowing, subchondral bony sclerosis, cystic changes, and osteophyte formation.

Nonsurgical management includes oral or topical nonsteroidal anti-inflammatory drugs and perhaps the use of intra-articular injections, such as steroids or viscosup-plementation.[43] Physical therapy to improve leg strength, flexibility, gait, and balance have been demonstrated to be as effective as nonsteroidal anti-inflammatory drugs for improved pain relief and function. Progressive resistance exercises, weight training in pain-free arcs of motion, and nonimpact exercises (eg, water aerobics and recumbent cycling) can help to maintain muscle tone and strength while improving endurance.[44] Surgical management of advanced cases often entails a total knee replacement.

Patellofemoral pain syndrome

Patellofemoral pain syndrome typically presents as a history of vague mild to moderate anterior knee pain exacerbated with prolonged periods of sitting (also referred to as the theater sign) or other activities that load the patellofemoral joint (such as squatting, ascending stairs, jogging, or running).[45] Most commonly seen in females in their 20 to 30s, patellofemoral pain syndrome is an umbrella term to capture all peripatellar or retropatellar pain in the absence of other pathologies. Overload of the anterior knee, abnormal patellar position or tracking, quadriceps dysfunction, and poor trunk and pelvic control are some factors that can cause the onset of pain associated with patellofemoral pain syndrome. The patient typically presents with anterior knee pain without a history of trauma and can occasionally present with a mild knee effusion. On physical examination, pain with a deep squat or tenderness of the patella with medial or lateral subluxation may lead to a diagnosis of patellofemoral pain syndrome.

Treatment typically consists of rest, activity modification, and physical therapy that focuses on hip and quadriceps strengthening.[46–48] Other interventions, such as patellar taping, foot orthoses, and braces, have limited evidence for long-term improvement of symptoms.[47]

Patellar tendinopathy

Patellar tendinopathy, also referred to as jumper's knee, represents a degenerative irritation and inflammation of the patellar tendon.[49] Symptoms typically consist of pain at the inferior pole of the patella what is exacerbated with activities that require cutting and changing direction. The pain is typically chronic in nature and not elicited by a single event, but repeated activities that involve repeated quadriceps activation, such as running, jumping, or going down stairs. Rarely is an effusion present. Pain is reproduced by resisted knee extension or with high loads such as a squat or jump. Pain on palpation of the patellar tendon is not a useful test because pain at this site is common and does not indicate that pain is from the tendon. Useful imaging modalities include ultrasound examination, which can demonstrate a thickened and hypervascular tendon, or MRI.

Treatment includes a period of rest followed by functional strengthening of the quadriceps, eccentric loading of the tendon, and correction of underlying biomechanical factors such as quadriceps and hamstring flexibility.[50–52] Platelet-rich plasma has demonstrated mixed results and evidence-based recommendations are mixed. Surgery may be indicated for patients with refractory symptoms despite attempts with conservative therapy.[50]

Anterior cruciate ligament injury

A tear of the ACL results from a rotational or hyperextension force applied during deceleration to the knee joint that overcomes the strength of the ligament. Most ACL tears occur with noncontact injuries and can be accompanied by a significant meniscal injury or in association with a tear of the MCL.[53] Patient's typically report sudden pain and giving way of the knee from a twisting or hyperextension type injury. One-third of patients report an audible pop when the ligament tears and athletes are typically unable to continue participation because of pain and/or instability.[54] If evaluated in the acute setting, an effusion from bleeding into the joint (hemarthrosis) is typically present. Physical examination findings, including a positive Lachman test

(81% sensitive) or the anterior drawer test (38% sensitive), can support suspicion for this injury type.[55] Every patient with a suspected ACL tear should undergo plain radiographs, which can show an effusion and possibly an avulsion fracture of the lateral capsular margin of the tibia (also referred to as a Segond fracture).[40] MRI is sensitive for detecting ACL tears and evaluating for other secondary injuries, including meniscal and collateral ligament damage.[56]

The initial treatment of an acute ACL injury includes rest, ice, and the use of crutches until the patient is able to ambulate with minimal pain and has regained normal range of motion. A knee immobilizer or range of motion brace may be used for comfort when necessary until pain subsides. Early range of motion exercises are important to maintain muscle strength and improve postoperative outcomes.[57] Definitive treatment of an ACL injury depends on the patient's age and desired level of activity and associated injuries. For young, active individuals, ACL reconstruction offers the best chance for a successful return to agility sports. Older or less active individuals may be treated with physical therapy aimed at controlling instability or provided ACL functional bracing to improve daily function. The risk of avoiding surgery for an ACL tear includes recurrent instability, subsequent meniscal tears, and degenerative disease of the knee.[58,59] The decision regarding ACL repair should be made in conjunction with an appropriately trained orthopedic surgeon to help determine benefits and risks, as well as ongoing monitoring of knee integrity if surgery is not pursued.

Medial collateral ligament injury
The MCL helps to stabilize the knee against valgus stresses and is typically injured by an abduction force without rotation, such as a clipping injury in football. These injuries can occur alone, but also can occur with a meniscal tear or an ACL or PCL tear. Patients typically report localized swelling or stiffness along the medial aspect of the, knee but do not report instability or mechanical symptoms, such as locking or popping, which are typically found in cruciate ligament or meniscal injuries.[60] The MCL may be tender along its entire course, from the medial femoral condyle to its insertion on the proximal tibia. Isolated tenderness at the most proximal or distal extend of the MCL may signify an avulsion-type injury. The examiner should apply valgus stress to the knee in full extension and at 30° of flexion to assess for knee stability or valgus laxity. The grade of injury can be determine by the degree of valgus joint space opening: no laxity (<5 mm medial joint opening) is considered a grade I tear, laxity with an endpoint (5–10 mm joint opening) a grade II tear, and laxity with no endpoint (>10 mm opening) a grade III tear.[61] Initial radiographs are typically negative in an MCL injury with exception to when there is an avulsion injury at the femoral origin of the MCL. MRI is sensitive for collateral ligament injuries and can also reveal other pathologies.[62]

Almost all MCL injuries can be treated without surgery.[63] Rest, ice, compression, and crutches can be used in the acute setting. For grade II and III injuries, a hinged knee brace with gradual increase in weight-bearing activity as well as several weeks to months of physical therapy are the mainstays of treatment.[64]

Meniscal injury
Meniscal injuries and tears cause disruption with the biomechanics of the knee, leading to varying degrees of symptoms, including locking, catching, or popping, as well as pain with twisting or squatting activities. Traumatic tears are typically followed by the insidious onset of knee swelling and stiffness over 2 to 3 days. In some cases, a large and unstable fragment of meniscus can become incarcerated in the knee joint, leading to a locked knee. The mechanical symptoms and degree of pain can wax and

wane, especially with degenerative meniscal tears seen in older individuals. The most common physical examination finding is tenderness over the medial or lateral joint line. During provocative testing, forced flexion and circumduction (internal and external rotation of the foot) frequently elicit pain on the side of the knee caused by the meniscal tear. The McMurray test is positive when the flexion-circumduction maneuver is also associated with a painful click.[65] The Thessaly test attempts to load the meniscus by having the patient stand on 1 leg with the knee flexed to 20° while internally and externally rotating the knee. Pain or a catching sensation signifies a positive test and has a reported sensitivity and specificity of 90% and 96%, respectively.[66] Plain radiographs may be indicated in patients with a history of trauma or effusion; however, MRI is more sensitive and specific to identify meniscal pathology.[40]

Surgery is indicated in patients who have a loss of range of motion or significant tears identified on MRI. Most degenerative meniscus injuries or small tears should be managed with a course of rest, nonsteroidal anti-inflammatories, and physical therapy focusing on functional motion and knee strengthening.[67]

Iliotibial band syndrome

The IT band is a dense, fibrous band of tissue that originates from the anterior superior iliac spine and extends down the lateral portion of the thigh, and inserts on the lateral tibia at the Gerdy's tubercle. IT band syndrome develops when the distal portion of the IT band rubs against the lateral femoral epicondyle, causing irritation and subsequent inflammation. This syndrome typically occurs with repetitive flexion and extension of the knee and is typically seen in long distance runners, cyclists, or athletes with underlying biomechanical predispositions, including genu varum, internal tibial rotation, and excessive foot protonation.[68] Pain is typically at the anterolateral aspect of the knee and worsens with running, especially downhill, or with cycling. Tenderness to direction palpation is most evident directly over the lateral femoral epicondyle, approximately 2 to 3 cm proximal to the lateral joint line. Noble compression and Ober tests may also help to confirm the diagnosis.[69] Imaging is often not required to diagnosis of IT band syndrome.

Treatment includes physical therapy focusing on improving hamstring and IT band flexibility as well as hip abductor strengthening.[70] Gait analysis or adjustment of biomechanics may be needed to correct underlying deficiencies that promoted the development of IT band syndrome.[71]

Popliteal (Baker's) cyst

A popliteal cyst, commonly referred to as a Baker's cyst, is the most common benign synovial cyst in the knee.[72] It develops in the popliteal bursa located at the posteromedial aspect of the knee joint. This bursa is normally very thin, communicates with the knee joint, and becomes more prominent when synovitis or trauma creates excessive joint fluid that tracks into the popliteal bursa. In adults, the mass almost always associated with a secondary intra-articular pathology, such as meniscal tears, ACL deficiencies, cartilage degeneration, and arthritis. Patients present with swelling or fullness in the popliteal fossa without a history of trauma. There may be associated pain and tenderness and these cysts can rupture spontaneously, causing severe calf pain and swelling.[73] The cysts are typically found between the medial head of the gastrocnemius muscle and the semimembranosus muscle. Although radiographs of the knee are typically negative, there may be an outline of the cyst of calcification of the cyst may be seen. MRI can be use if the diagnosis is uncertain. Ultrasound examination is also a reliable imaging modality to diagnose a Baker's cyst.[74]

These cysts are benign and typically treated with aspiration to help alleviate pain and pressure. This treatment may provide transient relief because the cyst can return. The cyst contents are typically quite gelatinous and may be difficult to aspirate. Treatment should also be directed at the cause of increased synovial fluid, typically degenerative arthritis or meniscal injuries, which can also be alleviated with intra-articular corticosteroid injections.[75] Ruptured popliteal cysts are treated symptomatically with minor analgesics, rest, and elevation.

Tibial apophysitis (Osgood-Schlatter disease)

Osgood-Schlatter disease is an overuse injury in a growing child that results from repetitive stress when a tightened quadriceps places excessive tension on apophysis of the tibial tuberosity during a period of rapid growth (approximately 11–13 years old).[76] Pain is typically exacerbated by running, jumping, and kneeling activities. Tenderness and swelling at the insertion of the patellar tendon into the tibial tubercle are common. Anteroposterior and lateral radiographs can show small spicules of heterotopic ossification anterior to the tibial tuberosity.

Symptoms are often controlled with use of ice after sports, nonsteroidal anti-inflammatories, and stretching exercises.[77] Reducing exercise and activity may permit healing and treat symptoms, but complete cessation of sport is not recommend because deconditioning increases the risk of recurrence or other injury. Immobilization is only required for severe or recalcitrant symptoms.[77] Activity may need to be modified for an average of 2 to 3 months for symptoms to improve in conjunction with a quadriceps strengthening program.[78] Some residual prominence of the tibial tubercle is common.

SUMMARY

Patients commonly consult their primary care providers for disorders related to the hip and knee. In this review, we discuss several of the most common presentations and diagnoses that a primary care provider may encounter when dealing with injuries of the hip and knee. This current burden highlights the need to provide appropriate, evidence-based care for patients, as well as to understand appropriate history questions, physical examination maneuvers, and imaging modalities to guide a practitioner to the correct diagnosis. Treatment for most musculoskeletal conditions typically involve rest, activity modification, ice, and anti-inflammatories, but understanding the role of physical therapy to correct underlying musculoskeletal weakness or biomechanical deficiencies, the role of injections, and consideration of surgery is important for those who do not respond to conservative care.

DISCLOSURE

The author has nothing to disclose.

REFERENCES

1. Tammareddi K, Morelli V, Reyes M. The athlete's hip and groin. Prim Care 2013; 40(2):313–33.
2. Christmas C, Crespo CJ, Franckowiak SC, et al. How common is hip pain among older adults? Results from the Third National Health and Nutrition Examination Survey. J Fam Pract 2002;51(4):345–8.
3. Ward RJ, Weissman BN, Kransdorf MJ, et al. ACR appropriateness criteria acute hip pain-suspected fracture. J Am Coll Radiol 2014;11(2):114–20.

4. Berquist TH, Dalinka MK, Alazraki N, et al. Chronic hip pain. American College of Radiology. ACR Appropriateness Criteria. Radiology 2000;215(Suppl):391–6.

5. Perdikakis E, Karachalios T, Katonis P, et al. Comparison of MR-arthrography and MDCT-arthrography for detection of labral and articular cartilage hip pathology. Skeletal Radiol 2011;40(11):1441–7.

6. Smith TO, Hilton G, Toms AP, et al. The diagnostic accuracy of acetabular labral tears using magnetic resonance imaging and magnetic resonance arthrography: a meta-analysis. Eur Radiol 2011;21(4):863–74.

7. Fransen M, McConnell S, Hernandez-Molina G, et al. Exercise for osteoarthritis of the hip. Cochrane Database Syst Rev 2014;(4):CD007912.

8. Zhang W, Moskowitz RW, Nuki G, et al. OARSI recommendations for the management of hip and knee osteoarthritis, part I: critical appraisal of existing treatment guidelines and systematic review of current research evidence. Osteoarthritis Cartilage 2007;15(9):981–1000.

9. Zhang W, Moskowitz RW, Nuki G, et al. OARSI recommendations for the management of hip and knee osteoarthritis, Part II: OARSI evidence-based, expert consensus guidelines. Osteoarthritis Cartilage 2008;16(2):137–62.

10. Kruse DW. Intraarticular cortisone injection for osteoarthritis of the hip. Is it effective? Is it safe? Curr Rev Musculoskelet Med 2008;1(3–4):227–33.

11. Banerjee P, McLean CR. Femoroacetabular impingement: a review of diagnosis and management. Curr Rev Musculoskelet Med 2011;4(1):23–32.

12. Philippon MJ, Maxwell RB, Johnston TL, et al. Clinical presentation of femoroacetabular impingement. Knee Surg Sports Traumatol Arthrosc 2007;15(8):1041–7.

13. Siebenrock KA, Kalbermatten DF, Ganz R. Effect of pelvic tilt on acetabular retroversion: a study of pelves from cadavers. Clin Orthop Relat Res 2003;407:241–8.

14. Ranawat AS, Schulz B, Baumbach SF, et al. Radiographic predictors of hip pain in femoroacetabular impingement. HSS J 2011;7(2):115–9.

15. Wall PD, Fernandez M, Griffin DR, et al. Nonoperative treatment for femoroacetabular impingement: a systematic review of the literature. PM R 2013;5(5): 418–26.

16. Krych AJ, Griffith TB, Hudgens JL, et al. Limited therapeutic benefits of intraarticular cortisone injection for patients with femoro-acetabular impingement and labral tear. Knee Surg Sports Traumatol Arthrosc 2014;22(4):750–5.

17. Griffin DR, Dickenson EJ, Wall PDH, et al. Hip arthroscopy versus best conservative care for the treatment of femoroacetabular impingement syndrome (UK FASHIoN): a multicentre randomised controlled trial. Lancet 2018;391(10136): 2225–35.

18. Mansell NS, Rhon DI, Meyer J, et al. Arthroscopic surgery or physical therapy for patients with femoroacetabular impingement syndrome: a randomized controlled trial with 2-year follow-up. Am J Sports Med 2018;46(6):1306–14.

19. McCarthy JC, Noble PC, Schuck MR, et al. The Otto E. Aufranc Award: the role of labral lesions to development of early degenerative hip disease. Clin Orthop Relat Res 2001;393:25–37.

20. Bharam S. Labral tears, extra-articular injuries, and hip arthroscopy in the athlete. Clin Sports Med 2006;25(2):279–92, ix.

21. Narvani AA, Tsiridis E, Kendall S, et al. A preliminary report on prevalence of acetabular labrum tears in sports patients with groin pain. Knee Surg Sports Traumatol Arthrosc 2003;11(6):403–8.

22. Theige M, David S. Nonsurgical treatment of acetabular labral tears. J Sport Rehabil 2018;27(4):380–4.

23. Harris JD. Hip labral repair: options and outcomes. Curr Rev Musculoskelet Med 2016;9(4):361–7.
24. Wolff AB, Grossman J. Management of the acetabular labrum. Clin Sports Med 2016;35(3):345–60.
25. Potalivo G, Bugiantella W. Snapping hip syndrome: systematic review of surgical treatment. Hip Int 2017;27(2):111–21.
26. Blankenbaker DG, De Smet AA, Keene JS. Sonography of the iliopsoas tendon and injection of the iliopsoas bursa for diagnosis and management of the painful snapping hip. Skeletal Radiol 2006;35(8):565–71.
27. Idjadi J, Meislin R. Symptomatic snapping hip: targeted treatment for maximum pain relief. Phys Sportsmed 2004;32(1):25–31.
28. Yen YM, Lewis CL, Kim YJ. Understanding and treating the snapping hip. Sports Med Arthrosc Rev 2015;23(4):194–9.
29. Johansson C, Ekenman I, Törnkvist H, et al. Stress fractures of the femoral neck in athletes. The consequence of a delay in diagnosis. Am J Sports Med 1990;18(5):524–8.
30. Bencardino JT, Stone TJ, Roberts CC, et al. ACR appropriateness criteria. J Am Coll Radiol 2017;14(5S):S293–306.
31. Clough TM. Femoral neck stress fracture: the importance of clinical suspicion and early review. Br J Sports Med 2002;36(4):308–9.
32. DeFranco MJ, Recht M, Schils J, et al. Stress fractures of the femur in athletes. Clin Sports Med 2006;25(1):89–103, ix.
33. Behrens SB, Deren ME, Matson A, et al. Stress fractures of the pelvis and legs in athletes: a review. Sports Health 2013;5(2):165–74.
34. Fearon AM, Scarvell JM, Neeman T, et al. Greater trochanteric pain syndrome: defining the clinical syndrome. Br J Sports Med 2013;47(10):649–53.
35. Fearon AM, Cook JL, Scarvell JM, et al. Greater trochanteric pain syndrome negatively affects work, physical activity and quality of life: a case control study. J Arthroplasty 2014;29(2):383–6.
36. Grimaldi A, Mellor R, Hodges P, et al. Gluteal tendinopathy: a review of mechanisms, assessment and management. Sports Med 2015;45(8):1107–19.
37. Grimaldi A, Mellor R, Nicolson P, et al. Utility of clinical tests to diagnose MRI-confirmed gluteal tendinopathy in patients presenting with lateral hip pain. Br J Sports Med 2017;51(6):519–24.
38. Lustenberger DP, Ng VY, Best TM, et al. Efficacy of treatment of trochanteric bursitis: a systematic review. Clin J Sport Med 2011;21(5):447–53.
39. Mellor R, Bennell K, Grimaldi A, et al. Education plus exercise versus corticosteroid injection use versus a wait and see approach on global outcome and pain from gluteal tendinopathy: prospective, single blinded, randomised clinical trial. Br J Sports Med 2018;52(22):1464–72.
40. Tuite MJ, Kransdorf MJ, Beaman FD, et al. ACR appropriateness criteria acute trauma to the knee. J Am Coll Radiol 2015;12(11):1164–72.
41. Cheung TC, Tank Y, Breederveld RS, et al. Diagnostic accuracy and reproducibility of the Ottawa Knee Rule vs the Pittsburgh Decision Rule. Am J Emerg Med 2013;31(4):641–5.
42. Fox MG, Chang EY, Amini B, et al. ACR appropriateness criteria. J Am Coll Radiol 2018;15(11S):S302–12.
43. Abbate LM, Jeffreys AS, Coffman CJ, et al. Demographic and clinical factors associated with nonsurgical osteoarthritis treatment among patients in outpatient clinics. Arthritis Care Res (Hoboken) 2018;70(8):1141–9.

44. Allen KD, Golightly YM, White DK. Gaps in appropriate use of treatment strategies in osteoarthritis. Best Pract Res Clin Rheumatol 2017;31(5):746–59.
45. Crossley KM, Stefanik JJ, Selfe J, et al. Patellofemoral pain consensus statement from the 4th International Patellofemoral Pain Research Retreat, Manchester. Part 1: terminology, definitions, clinical examination, natural history, patellofemoral osteoarthritis and patient-reported outcome measures. Br J Sports Med 2016; 50(14):839–43.
46. Crossley KM, Vicenzino B, Lentzos J, et al. Exercise, education, manual-therapy and taping compared to education for patellofemoral osteoarthritis: a blinded, randomised clinical trial. Osteoarthritis Cartilage 2015;23(9):1457–64.
47. Collins NJ, Barton CJ, van Middelkoop M, et al. Consensus statement on exercise therapy and physical interventions (orthoses, taping and manual therapy) to treat patellofemoral pain: recommendations from the 5th International Patellofemoral Pain Research Retreat, Gold Coast, Australia, 2017. Br J Sports Med 2018; 52(18):1170–8.
48. Barton CJ, Lack S, Hemmings S, et al. The 'Best Practice Guide to Conservative Management of Patellofemoral Pain': incorporating level 1 evidence with expert clinical reasoning. Br J Sports Med 2015;49(14):923–34.
49. Wilson JJ, Best TM. Common overuse tendon problems: a review and recommendations for treatment. Am Fam Physician 2005;72(5):811–8.
50. Schwartz A, Watson JN, Hutchinson MR. Patellar tendinopathy. Sports Health 2015;7(5):415–20.
51. Gaida JE, Cook J. Treatment options for patellar tendinopathy: critical review. Curr Sports Med Rep 2011;10(5):255–70.
52. Everhart JS, Cole D, Sojka JH, et al. Treatment options for patellar tendinopathy: a systematic review. Arthroscopy 2017;33(4):861–72.
53. Griffin LY, Agel J, Albohm MJ, et al. Noncontact anterior cruciate ligament injuries: risk factors and prevention strategies. J Am Acad Orthop Surg 2000;8(3):141–50.
54. Wagemakers HP, Luijsterburg PA, Boks SS, et al. Diagnostic accuracy of history taking and physical examination for assessing anterior cruciate ligament lesions of the knee in primary care. Arch Phys Med Rehabil 2010;91(9):1452–9.
55. Benjaminse A, Gokeler A, van der Schans CP. Clinical diagnosis of an anterior cruciate ligament rupture: a meta-analysis. J Orthop Sports Phys Ther 2006; 36(5):267–88.
56. Crawford R, Walley G, Bridgman S, et al. Magnetic resonance imaging versus arthroscopy in the diagnosis of knee pathology, concentrating on meniscal lesions and ACL tears: a systematic review. Br Med Bull 2007;84:5–23.
57. Spindler KP, Wright RW. Clinical practice. Anterior cruciate ligament tear. N Engl J Med 2008;359(20):2135–42.
58. Lohmander LS, Englund PM, Dahl LL, et al. The long-term consequence of anterior cruciate ligament and meniscus injuries: osteoarthritis. Am J Sports Med 2007;35(10):1756–69.
59. Neuman P, Englund M, Kostogiannis I, et al. Prevalence of tibiofemoral osteoarthritis 15 years after nonoperative treatment of anterior cruciate ligament injury: a prospective cohort study. Am J Sports Med 2008;36(9):1717–25.
60. Kastelein M, Wagemakers HP, Luijsterburg PA, et al. Assessing medial collateral ligament knee lesions in general practice. Am J Med 2008;121(11):982–8.e2.
61. Rasenberg EI, Lemmens JA, van Kampen A, et al. Grading medial collateral ligament injury: comparison of MR imaging and instrumented valgus-varus laxity test-device. A prospective double-blind patient study. Eur J Radiol 1995;21(1): 18–24.

62. Kurzweil PR, Kelley ST. Physical examination and imaging of the medial collateral ligament and posteromedial corner of the knee. Sports Med Arthrosc Rev 2006; 14(2):67–73.
63. Derscheid GL, Garrick JG. Medial collateral ligament injuries in football. Nonoperative management of grade I and grade II sprains. Am J Sports Med 1981;9(6): 365–8.
64. Reider B. Medial collateral ligament injuries in athletes. Sports Med 1996;21(2): 147–56.
65. Solomon DH, Simel DL, Bates DW, et al. The rational clinical examination. Does this patient have a torn meniscus or ligament of the knee? Value of the physical examination. JAMA 2001;286(13):1610–20.
66. Karachalios T, Hantes M, Zibis AH, et al. Diagnostic accuracy of a new clinical test (the Thessaly test) for early detection of meniscal tears. J Bone Joint Surg Am 2005;87(5):955–62.
67. Kise NJ, Risberg MA, Stensrud S, et al. Exercise therapy versus arthroscopic partial meniscectomy for degenerative meniscal tear in middle aged patients: randomised controlled trial with two year follow-up. Br J Sports Med 2016;50(23): 1473–80.
68. Orchard JW, Fricker PA, Abud AT, et al. Biomechanics of iliotibial band friction syndrome in runners. Am J Sports Med 1996;24(3):375–9.
69. Strauss EJ, Kim S, Calcei JG, et al. Iliotibial band syndrome: evaluation and management. J Am Acad Orthop Surg 2011;19(12):728–36.
70. Fredericson M, Cookingham CL, Chaudhari AM, et al. Hip abductor weakness in distance runners with iliotibial band syndrome. Clin J Sport Med 2000;10(3): 169–75.
71. Fredericson M, Wolf C. Iliotibial band syndrome in runners: innovations in treatment. Sports Med 2005;35(5):451–9.
72. Handy JR. Popliteal cysts in adults: a review. Semin Arthritis Rheum 2001;31(2): 108–18.
73. Katz RS, Zizic TM, Arnold WP, et al. The pseudothrombophlebitis syndrome. Medicine (Baltimore) 1977;56(2):151–64.
74. Wisniewski SJ, Murthy N, Smith J. Ultrasound evaluation of Baker cysts: diagnosis and management. PM R 2012;4(7):533–7.
75. Acebes JC, Sánchez-Pernaute O, Díaz-Oca A, et al. Ultrasonographic assessment of Baker's cysts after intra-articular corticosteroid injection in knee osteoarthritis. J Clin Ultrasound 2006;34(3):113–7.
76. Kujala UM, Kvist M, Heinonen O. Osgood-Schlatter's disease in adolescent athletes. Retrospective study of incidence and duration. Am J Sports Med 1985; 13(4):236–41.
77. Bloom OJ, Mackler L, Barbee J. Clinical inquiries. What is the best treatment for Osgood-Schlatter disease? J Fam Pract 2004;53(2):153–6.
78. Wall EJ. Osgood-Schlatter disease: practical treatment for a self-limiting condition. Phys Sportsmed 1998;26(3):29–34.

Approaching Foot and Ankle Injuries in the Ambulatory Setting

Andrew W. Albano Jr, DO[a,b,]*, Vicki Nelson, MD, PhD[b,c]

KEYWORDS

- Achilles tendon rupture • Ankle sprain • Syndesmotic injury
- Metatarsal stress fracture • Jones fracture • Plantar fasciitis • Sports medicine

KEY POINTS

- Because foot and ankle pain is a commonly encountered complaint in the ambulatory setting, primary care physicians need to familiarize themselves with their potential causes.
- Understanding the key points of the history and physical examination can help the primary care physician quickly narrow the differential diagnosis, use the appropriate imaging modality, and implement the correct treatment plan.
- The utilization of special examination maneuvers can help in identifying the likely cause of foot and ankle pain.

EVALUATION OF FOOT AND ANKLE INJURIES
History

In addressing the acutely injured foot or ankle, attention should be paid to gathering an appropriate history and completing a methodical physical examination. At the time of evaluation, the following questions should be addressed[1]:

- When and where did this injury occur?
- How was the foot positioned at the time of injury?
- In which direction was the ankle joint stressed?
- Immediately following injury, what was the patient's weight-bearing ability?
- Were any audible sounds appreciated at the time of injury?
- What is the degree of pain and disability the patient has experienced since injury?
- Has there been any swelling or discoloration of the foot, ankle, or lower leg?
- Were there any prior injuries or surgeries to the affected lower limb?

[a] Quality & Medical Affairs, Department of Family Medicine, Prisma Health, 877 West Faris Road, Greenville, SC 29605, USA; [b] University of South Carolina School of Medicine–Greenville, Greenville, SC, USA; [c] Department of Family Medicine, Prisma Health, 877 West Faris Road, Greenville, SC 29605, USA
* Corresponding author. 877 West Faris Road, Greenville, SC 29605.
E-mail address: Drew.Albano@prismahealth.org
Twitter: @DrDrewAlbano (A.W.A.)

Prim Care Clin Office Pract 47 (2020) 133–145
https://doi.org/10.1016/j.pop.2019.10.007
0095-4543/20/© 2019 Elsevier Inc. All rights reserved.
primarycare.theclinics.com

- Has treatment been previously sought?
- Has any treatment been attempted (eg, ice, compression, anti-inflammatory medications)?

Physical Examination

At the onset of the physical examination, gait and weight-bearing status should be assessed.[1-3] Exposing the affected area allows for a thorough visual inspection with appreciation for swelling, ecchymosis, and/or compromise to the overlying soft tissue. Commonly, diffuse swelling occurs with foot, ankle, and lower leg injuries, obscuring anatomic landmarks and confounding injury localization.[1-3] Palpation can help to isolate an area or areas suspicious for bony injury[2]; however, the usefulness of palpation may also be limited by soft tissue swelling and patient discomfort. Pain localized along the anterior or posterior ankle joint may indicate capsular or intraarticular involvement. Incorporating information obtained from the gathered history can facilitate the necessity of special examination maneuvers (**Table 1**) to address specific areas of concern.[4]

Imaging

Radiography

Developed in an effort to reduce unnecessary ankle radiography, the Ottawa Foot and Ankle Rules (**Fig. 1**) have been found to have high sensitivity with low specificity.[5,6] Per these rules, it is recommended that ankle radiographs be obtained if a patient presents with the following[7]:

- Pain at the posterior edge or tip (distal 6 cm) of either malleoli
- An inability to bear weight immediately after injury *and* for 4 steps in the emergency department.

It is recommended that foot radiographs be obtained if a patient presents with the following:

- Pain in the midfoot and
- Inability to bear weight immediately after injury *or* has bony tenderness at the navicular or the base of the fifth metatarsal.

Magnetic resonance imaging

In certain clinical presentations, MRI can be beneficial in confirming the diagnosis, but routine MRI of an acutely injured foot or ankle is not recommended.[8]

Ultrasonography

As a cost-effective and radiation-free imaging modality, ultrasound provides the ability to complete dynamic assessments and conduct a real-time evaluation of the injury.[9,10]

ANKLE INJURIES

The ankle is the most frequently injured joint,[1,2,11] and subsequently, a significant source of morbidity and long-term disability.[12] Delineating between the various causes for ankle pain can pose a diagnostic challenge in the ambulatory setting. Familiarity with commonly encountered ankle injuries can aid the primary care clinician in their approach to this clinical presentation.

Anatomy

The ankle comprises 2 joints: The articulations of the distal fibula, distal tibia, and the talus form the talocrural joint, and the articulation of the talus and the calcaneus

Table 1
Special examination maneuvers of the foot and ankle

Test	Description	Positive Finding	Conditions Associated with Positive Finding
Thompson test (Simmonds test)	With the patient prone, place the patient's ipsilateral foot over the edge of the examination table and squeeze the calf	Absence of a passive flexion of the ipsilateral foot	Achilles tendon rupture
Anterior drawer test	With the patient supine, and the patient's foot in slight plantarflexion, brace the anterior shin with 1 hand and translate the heel anteriorly with the other hand. Comparison is made to the contralateral side	Laxity and absence of a firm end point	Lateral ankle sprain • ATFL rupture • Possible CFL rupture
Talar tilt test	With the patient seated or supine and the tibia and fibula stabilized, the ipsilateral foot is inverted and everted. Comparison is made to the contralateral side	Laxity and/or pain	Lateral ankle sprain • ATFL rupture • CFL rupture
Squeeze test	With the patient seated or supine, compress the patient's lower leg about midway up the calf	Pain in the area of the distal tibiofibular and interosseous ligaments with proximal calf compression	Syndesmotic injury
External rotation test (syndesmotic stress test)	With the patient seated on the examination table and the knee flexed over the edge of the table, the proximal lower leg is stabilized while the foot is grasped (plantar surface/heel) and dorsiflexed. The foot is then externally rotated	Pain in the area of the distal tibiofibular and interosseous ligaments	Syndesmotic injury
Calcaneal squeeze test	With the knee flexed at 90°, the examiner squeezes the sides of the calcaneus	Pain at the site	Calcaneal stress fracture

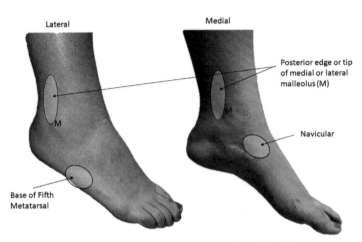

Fig. 1. The Anatomic Landmarks of the Ottawa Foot and Ankle Rules.

forms the subtalar joint.[2] The syndesmotic ligaments along with the interosseous membrane provide stability between the fibula and the tibia.[1,2,12] The anterior-inferior tibiofibular ligament attaches the distal anterior tibia to the distal anterior fibula, and the posterior-inferior tibiofibular ligament attaches the distal posterior tibia to the distal posterior fibula.[2] Syndesmotic incompetence causes instability, primarily in the anterior to posterior direction.[2,12] The mortise created from the bony articulations of the ankle allows for plantarflexion and dorsiflexion of the foot. The subtalar joint allows for eversion and inversion of the foot. Inversion injuries typically yield compromise to the anterior talofibular ligament (ATFL), and less often, the calcaneofibular ligament (CFL).[1] Rarely, the posterior talofibular ligament may also be subject to injury.

Motion through the ankle joint is controlled by 4 groups of muscles. Laterally, eversion and a portion of plantarflexion are controlled by the peroneal musculature originating from the fibula and inserting into the base of the fifth metatarsal (peroneus brevis) and the base of the first metatarsal (peroneus longus).[1,2] Medially, the posterior tibialis allows for inversion of the midfoot, whereas the flexor digitorum longus and flexor hallucis longus control flexion of the digits.[1,2] Anteriorly, the anterior tibialis, originating from the medial tibia, inserts onto the plantar aspect of the first metatarsal and navicular, controlling dorsiflexion and inversion.[1,2] The extensor digitorum attaches to the phalanges from the fibula, controlling digit extension. Posteriorly, the confluence of the gastrocnemius and soleus muscles forms the Achilles tendon, inserting on the calcaneus and providing plantarflexion of the foot.[1,2]

Common Ankle Injuries

Ankle sprains
Lateral ankle sprains typically result from an inversion of the plantarflexed foot, often occurring during athletic activity, or from walking or running on uneven surfaces.[13,14] Significant swelling and ecchymosis can be observed following injury. Competency of the ATFL can be assessed with the anterior drawer test (**Fig. 2**). The competency of the CFL can be assessed with completing the talar tilt test (**Fig. 3**).[14] The Ottawa Ankle Rules aid in determining the utility of radiographic imaging.[6,7] MRI may be useful in the evaluation of persistent ankle pain in the absence of significant radiographic findings. MRI has high sensitivity and specificity for visualizing occult fractures, tendon

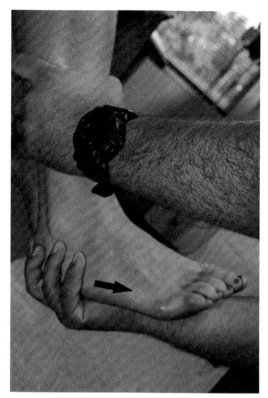

Fig. 2. Competency of the ATFL can be assessed with the anterior drawer test. The arrows indicate the direction the examiner moves the patient's foot to conduct the specific examination maneuver.

tears, or talar dome osteochondral defects and can aid in determining the extent of ligamentous injury.[13]

Treatment of ankle sprains varies according to the severity of injury. For lateral ankle sprains, rest, ice, compression, and elevation (RICE) has been endorsed as first-line treatment,[15] but research has found this treatment approach to be insufficient.[13] For more severe injuries, casting, taping, bracing,[16] or controlled ankle motion (CAM)-boot immobilization may be used. Treatment is usually continued until the patient is asymptomatic, but immobilization should not be continued for more than 10 days.[13] After an initial period of immobilization, therapy traditionally focuses on ankle range of motion, strengthening, and proprioceptive exercises,[17] although the benefit compared with usual care may not yield substantial differences in functional outcomes 6 months following injury.[18] For recurrent ankle sprains with minimal trauma and symptoms of ankle instability, surgical evaluation for the repair or reconstruction of the ATFL may offer relief.[13]

Achilles tendinopathy

Achilles tendinopathy is multifactorial,[19,20] resulting from both intrinsic (eg, diabetes mellitus) and extrinsic factors (eg, overuse). On presentation, weakness, pain, and swelling of the tendon are often observed.[21] MRI can be used to assess the integrity of the tendon, and neovascularization of the tendon can be assessed with power

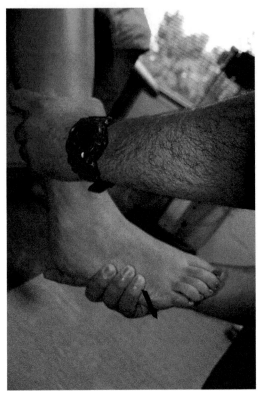

Fig. 3. The competency of the CFL can be assessed with completing the talar tilt test. The arrows indicate the direction the examiner moves the patient's foot to conduct the specific examination maneuver.

Doppler ultrasonography.[22] Acutely, first-line treatment should include rest, nonsteroidal anti-inflammatory drugs (NSAIDs) for analgesia, and physical therapy with a focus on eccentric exercises.[23] With symptom improvement, a graded return to previous function is recommended. Prolonged immobilization should be avoided.[20] There is currently no gold standard for management of this condition should conservative measures fail; however, minimally invasive surgery has shown promise.[22] Research exploring the benefit of ultrasound, prolotherapy, extracorporeal shockwave therapy, and low-level laser therapy is currently ongoing.[22] Because of the high risk of tendon damage and rupture, corticosteroid injection is not recommended.[20] Failure of conservative management may result in the need for surgical intervention.

Rupture of the Achilles tendon
Rupture of the Achilles tendon is often a result of explosive plantarflexion, as seen with sprinting or jumping, or with maximal dorsiflexion.[24] At the time of injury, patients often complain of the sensation of being struck on the posterior lower leg. It is important to exclude recent fluoroquinolone usage, a history significant for inflammatory disorders, and/or any introduction of local corticosteroids into the surrounding soft tissue.[25] Significant swelling and ecchymosis proximal to the calcaneus are often appreciated on examination. In addition, there may be a defect present at the site of tendon rupture.[24] Patients usually are unable to plantarflex the affected side when compared with the

contralateral limb. A positive Thompson test is suggestive of a complete rupture of the Achilles tendon.[25] Ultrasonography can be helpful in dynamic evaluation of the Achilles tendon.[9] Alternatively, MRI of the Achilles tendon can confirm the diagnosis if there is uncertainty and has utility in surgical planning.[24] Plain radiographs can be obtained to exclude an alternative diagnosis but cannot provide direct visualization of the tendon. Treatment approaches for the acute rupture of the Achilles tendon are debatable.[26] Consensus opinion does not favor casting as a superior treatment approach to a CAM boot with heel lift. However, research suggests that treatment with functional bracing and early range of motion therapy yields rerupture rates approaching those of surgical treatment.[24,27,28]

Talar osteochondral lesions

Osteochondral lesions of the talar dome are usually the result of a twisting injury of the ankle, the result of a fall, or from a vascular insult.[14,29] Pain and swelling of the ankle are commonly encountered on examination, with some patients reporting instability or mechanical symptoms, such as catching or locking.[29,30] Lesions can be missed on plain radiographs; therefore, localization and characterization of a lesion are best achieved via single-photon emission computed tomography-computed tomography (CT) scan or MRI scan.[30] Nonoperative treatment with NSAIDs, activity modification, and immobilization in a non-weight-bearing splint or cast can be successful in cases involving a small defect and/or nondisplaced bony fragment.[14,29,30] Surgical intervention is preferred for large defects (>1.5 cm), or when an osseous component is needed to achieve bony fixation.[14,29]

Peroneal tendinosis/peroneal subluxation

Peroneal tendinosis can be difficult to distinguish from lateral ankle ligamentous injury, and it is often overlooked as the source for lateral ankle pain and dysfunction.[31] It is often associated with ankle instability. Assessment of foot type (pes cavus/pes planus), palpation of the tendons in the retromalleolar groove, as well as testing of the lateral ankle ligaments should be completed during the physical examination.[31] With peroneal subluxation, forceful dorsiflexion of the ankle coupled with hindfoot inversion and contraction of the peroneal tendons causes disruption of the superior peroneal retinaculum.[31] Risk factors include a convex retromalleolar groove and a varus heel often yielding instability, and tendon pathologic condition. Ultrasound and MRI are the preferred imaging modalities for dynamic and static assessment of tendon integrity and function.[31,32] Conservative treatment consists of NSAIDs, rest, activity modification, and orthoses: lateral forefoot posting in mild cases.[31] For refractory cases, benefit may be seen with immobilization in a short-leg cast or CAM boot walker for 6 weeks.[31] For patients with peroneal tendon subluxation, conservative management tends to be insufficient with surgical intervention often required for definitive treatment.[31]

Syndesmotic injury (high ankle sprain)

Syndesmotic injuries typically occur as a result of an eversion and external rotation injury of the planted foot.[33] This injury may be difficult to diagnose. Squeezing the proximal tibia and fibula together (squeeze test) at the level of the calf places stress on the distal syndesmotic ligaments, whereas the external rotation stress test externally rotates the foot as the knee is stabilized in flexion.[33] Pain over the distal syndesmotic ligaments for either maneuver would be considered a positive finding. Syndesmotic injuries often accompany fractures. Fractures of the medial malleolus or ruptures of the deltoid ligament may be associated with syndesmotic injuries.[33] Radiographs of the tibia, fibula, and ankle joint should be obtained to rule out a fracture, including a Maisonneuve fracture of the proximal fibula.[34] In the absence of fracture, widening of the bony articulations can be suggestive of a syndesmotic injury.[33,35] MRI can aid with the diagnosis as well as in recognizing the presence of an occult fracture.[36] Patients with symptoms of a syndesmotic injury, with no evidence of radiographic widening, can be treated nonoperatively.[36] These injuries require a prolonged recovery in comparison to lateral ankle sprains.[33] For minor sprains, patients can be placed in a cast or air walking boot. Alternatively, patients can be made non-weight-bearing for approximately 3 to 4 weeks and then begin protected weight-bearing and therapy.[36] For a more severe injury, including medial malleolus or distal fibula fracture, or gross widening of the syndesmosis, surgical evaluation is recommended.[33,36]

Ankle arthropathy/posttraumatic ankle arthritis

Osteoarthritis of the tibiotalar joint is often posttraumatic[11,37] or degenerative in nature. Pain, swelling, and stiffness in the anterior ankle are common findings,[37] as is a history significant for trauma. On examination, a loss of ankle range of motion is common, and some patients may have a gait disturbance. Plain radiographs can confirm the presence and severity of osteoarthritis: joint space narrowing, osteophytes, subchondral sclerosis, and/or cysts.[38] Nonoperative treatment aims to curb pain with oral NSAIDs, modify activity level, address body habitus, and/or introduce corticosteroid via intraarticular injection.[37] Custom ankle-foot orthoses may be of benefit.[37] Research on early detection of posttraumatic osteoarthritis and the utility of viscosupplementation is ongoing,[39] but curative pharmaceutical and surgical interventions remain limited.[11] Arthroscopic ankle arthrodesis is a preferred surgical option for patients with refractory symptoms.[40]

FOOT INJURIES

Because it bears the entire weight of the body, the foot is under a great deal of stress and is prone to injury.[41] Foot injuries can be debilitating because of restrictions in ambulation and often require prolonged recovery periods. A thorough understanding of the anatomy is essential to definitively diagnose and treat the underlying problem effectively.

Anatomy

The foot can be thought of in 3 regions: the hindfoot consisting of the talus and calcaneus; the midfoot comprising the tarsal bones; and the forefoot housing the remaining metatarsals and phalanges. Foot anatomy can vary significantly among individuals with regards to length, width, curvature, and arch (eg, pes planus, pes cavus). Accessory ossicles commonly encountered in the foot include the os trigonum, os peroneum, and os naviculare.

In daily activities and most athletic pursuits, the foot serves an important role: serving as a rigid base for standing and to absorb the impact of body weight during gait. Stability during walking and activity requires several ligamentous structures to remain intact, notably the Lisfranc ligament at the tarsometatarsal junction. The posterior tibialis tendon serves an important role in stabilizing the plantar surface and maintaining the absorptive integrity of the plantar arch.

Common Foot Injuries

Fifth metatarsal fractures

Fractures of the fifth metatarsal are one of the most common foot injuries.[42] Injury is usually sustained as a direct blow to the lateral foot or through an inversion injury.

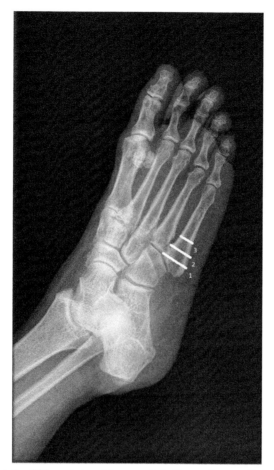

Fig. 4. Fractures at the fifth metatarsal base and shaft are often well visualized with plain radiographs for a definitive diagnosis.

Patients often present with considerable pain, tenderness, and swelling localized to the area of fracture. Axial loading of the metatarsal may be used in diagnosis because this should not produce pain in the absence of fracture. Fractures at the fifth metatarsal base and shaft are often well visualized with plain radiographs for a definitive diagnosis (**Fig. 4**).

Treatment of fifth metatarsal fractures depends on the location of injury. A nondisplaced styloid avulsion fracture may be managed nonoperatively by the primary care physician.[43] A firm-soled shoe or CAM boot may be used to allow weight-bearing as tolerated with a healing time of 6 to 8 weeks. Use of ice or anti-inflammatory medications can be used for analgesia. Displaced fractures (>3 mm) and fractures in the remaining length of the fifth metatarsal should be referred for specialist evaluation.[43] The Jones fracture, a fracture at the metaphyseal-diaphyseal junction, is slow to heal because of poor blood supply. These fractures could benefit from surgical consultation and consideration of fixation because they require prolonged immobilization (2–3 months) to heal.[43] The fifth metatarsal diaphysis is particularly susceptible to stress reaction or stress fracture. These injuries often result from repetitive pivoting activities and are also slow to heal. Healing requires strict non-weight-bearing and often takes 20 weeks for healing without surgical fixation.[43]

Plantar fasciitis/plantar heel pain

The plantar heel is the most common site of hindfoot pain. Although plantar fasciitis is the most common cause of plantar heel pain, it must be differentiated from alternative diagnoses, such as heel fat pad atrophy or calcaneal stress fracture. The plantar fascia is a thick, fibrous tissue attaching to the medial aspect of the plantar calcaneus. Patients with plantar fasciitis describe pain most often at the medial aspect of the calcaneus at the central plantar fascia insertion. Pain is characteristically most severe with the first steps in the morning and gradually improves with activity. Diagnosis is often made on the basis of clinical evaluation. Radiographs may reveal spurring at the plantar calcaneus, but this finding is not present in all cases. Ultrasound may be helpful to evaluate for heel fat pad atrophy, which often presents similarly with diffuse tenderness on the central calcaneus. A calcaneal squeeze test can be used to rule out calcaneal stress fracture. CT or MRI may be helpful if the diagnosis remains equivocal because calcaneal stress fractures are often not visualized on plain film.[44]

Treatment of plantar fasciitis is typically prolonged, and symptoms may take 6 to 12 months to resolve. Initial treatment is primarily symptomatic and may include modification of shoe wear, changes in activity, stretching, ice, and NSAIDs. Patients with debilitating symptoms may benefit from a period of immobilization or night splinting. Injection therapies, such as corticosteroid or autologous blood products (eg, platelet-rich plasma), may be considered an adjuvant therapy.[45,46] Newer modalities, such as extracorporeal shockwave therapy, may be useful in recalcitrant cases.[47,48]

Metatarsal stress fractures

Diagnosis of a metatarsal stress fracture is often based on clinical suspicion and a history of repetitive impact over time with insufficient rest or nutrition as bone resorption outpaces bone regeneration. A detailed history of training load, such as intensity, mileage, or frequency of activity, should be obtained.[49] Pain is often insidious in onset, worsened with activity, and initially improves with rest. A history of trauma may be seen in cases of acute fracture in an area of stress-related weakening but is not necessary for diagnosis. Pain and swelling are often well localized over the affected area of the metatarsal. Periosteal thickening or a true fracture line may be seen on radiographs; however, it may take 2 weeks or more from the onset of pain for visualization on plain film. If a definitive diagnosis is desired more readily, MRI or bone scan may be helpful early in the course.

Treatment generally consists of adequate rest and sufficient time for healing. The patient should be restricted from activity and non-weight-bearing or with protected ambulation, such as in a CAM boot. Evaluation for Relative Energy Deficiency states should be considered, particularly in patients with a history of prior stress fracture or stress fractures that show delayed healing.[50]

Posterior tibialis tendon dysfunction

The posterior tibialis is a primary stabilizer of the longitudinal arch, coursing behind the medial malleolus and inserting at the navicular and medial cuneiform. Tendon dysfunction is common in individuals with pes planus but is also often seen in individuals presenting with acquired arch collapse.[51] Pain often develops gradually and is localized to the medial ankle or foot. Passive stretch of the posterior tibialis tendon in eversion and active firing in resisted inversion frequently reproduce symptoms.

Treatment consists of RICE, anti-inflammatory medication, activity modification, modification of shoe wear, and/or orthotic shoe inserts.[52] Manual therapy and therapeutic ultrasound may also be helpful if symptoms persist.

DISCLOSURE

The authors have nothing to disclose.

REFERENCES

1. Birrer R. Ankle injuries and the family physician. J Am Board Fam Pract 1988;1(4): 274–81.
2. Harmon K. The ankle examination. Prim Care 2004;31(Issue 4):1025–37.
3. Young C, Niedfelt M, Morris G, et al. Clinical examination of the foot and ankle. Prim Care 2005;32(Issue 1):105–32.
4. Schwieterman B, Haas D, Columber K, et al. Diagnostic accuracy of physical examination tests of the ankle/foot complex: a systematic review. Int J Sports Phys Ther 2013;8(4):416–26.
5. Pires R, Pereira A, Abreu-E-Silva G, et al. Ottawa Ankle Rules and subjective surgeon perception to evaluate radiograph necessity following foot and ankle sprain. Ann Med Health Sci Res 2014;4(3):432–5.
6. Bachmann LM, Kolb E, Koller MT, et al. Accuracy of Ottawa Ankle Rules to exclude fracture of the ankle and mid-foot: a systematic review. BMJ 2003; 326:417.
7. Stiell IG, Greenberg GH, McKnight RD, et al. A study to develop clinical decision rules for the use of radiography in acute ankle injuries. Ann Emerg Med 1992;21: 384–90.
8. Tocci SL, Madom IA, Bradley MP, et al. The diagnostic value of MRI in foot and ankle surgery. Foot Ankle Int 2007;28(2):166–8.
9. Park J, Lee S, Kim S, et al. Ultrasonography of the ankle joint. Ultrasonography 2017;36(4):321–35.
10. Beard NM, Grouse RP. Current ultrasound application in the foot and ankle. Orthop Clin North Am 2018;49(1):109–21.
11. Carbone A, Rodeo S. Review of current understanding of post traumatic osteoarthritis resulting from sports injuries. J Orthop Res 2017;35:397–405.
12. Reissig J, Bitterman A, Lee S. Common foot and ankle injuries: what not to miss and how best to manage. J Am Osteopath Assoc 2017;117:98–104.
13. Vuurberg G, Hoorntje A, Wink LM, et al. Diagnosis, treatment and prevention of ankle sprains: update of an evidence-based clinical guideline. Br J Sports Med 2018;52:956.
14. Gill L, Klingele K. Management of foot and ankle injuries in pediatric and adolescent athletes: a narrative review. Orthop Res Rev 2018;10:19–30.
15. Paulson C, Hemphill B, Whitworth JD, et al. Clinical inquiry: how can we minimize recurrent ankle sprains. J Fam Pract 2011;60(12):759–60.
16. Barelds I, van den Broek AG, Huisstede BMA. Ankle bracing is effective for primary and secondary prevention of acute ankle injuries in athletes: a systematic review and meta-analyses. Sports Med 2018;48(12):2775–84.
17. Doherty C, Bleakley C, Delahunt E, et al. Treatment and prevention of acute and recurrent ankle sprain: an overview of systematic reviews with meta-analysis. Br J Sports Med 2017;51:113–25.

18. Brison RJ, Day AG, Pelland L, et al. Effect of early supervised physiotherapy on recovery from acute ankle sprain: randomised controlled trial. BMJ 2016;355: i5650.

19. Maffulli N, Florio A, Osti L, et al. Achilles tendinopathy. JBJS Rev 2014;2(9):1–11.

20. Li HY, Hua YH. Achilles tendinopathy: current concepts about the basic science and clinical treatments. Biomed Res Int 2016;2016:6492597.

21. Chimenti RL, Cychosz CC, Hall MM, et al. Current concepts review update: insertional Achilles tendinopathy. Foot Ankle Int 2017;38(10):1160–9.

22. Pearce CJ, Tan A. Non-insertional Achilles tendinopathy. EFORT Open Rev 2016; 1(11):383–90.

23. McCormack JR, Underwood FB, Slaven EJ, et al. Eccentric exercise versus eccentric exercise and soft tissue treatment (Astym) in the management of insertional Achilles tendinopathy. Sports Health 2016;8(3):230–7.

24. Egger AC, Berkowitz MJ. Achilles tendon injuries. Curr Rev Musculoskelet Med 2017;10(1):72–80.

25. Saleh A, Sadeghpour R, Munyak J. Foot and ankle update. Prim Care 2013;40: 383–406.

26. Maffulli G, Buono AD, Richards P, et al. Conservative, minimally invasive and open surgical repair for management of acute ruptures of the Achilles tendon: a clinical and functional retrospective study. Muscles Ligaments Tendons J 2017;7(1):46–52.

27. Miller L, Spittler J, Khodaee M, et al. FPIN's clinical inquiries. Management of acute Achilles tendon rupture. Am Fam Physician 2015;91(11):794–800.

28. Willits K, Annuziato A, Bryant D, et al. Operative versus nonoperative treatment of acute Achilles tendon ruptures: a multicenter randomized trial using accelerated functional rehabilitation. J Bone Joint Surg Am 2010;92(17):2767–75.

29. Rubin A, Sallis R. Evaluation and diagnosis of ankle injuries. Am Fam Physician 1996;54:5.

30. Rungprai C, Tennant JN, Gentry RD, et al. Management of osteochondral lesions of the talar dome. Open Orthop J 2017;11:743–61.

31. Davda K, Malhotra K, O'Donnell P, et al. Peroneal tendon disorders. EFFORT Open Rev 2017;2(6):281–92.

32. Molini L, Bianchi S. US in peroneal tendon tear. J Ultrasound 2014;17(2):125–34.

33. Yuen CP, Lui TH. Distal tibiofibular syndesmosis: anatomy, biomechanics, injury and management. Open Orthop J 2017;11:670–7.

34. Schnetzke M, Vetter SY, Beisemann N, et al. Management of syndesmotic injuries: what is the evidence? World J Orthop 2016;7(11):718–25.

35. Porter DA, Jaggers RR, Barnes AF, et al. Optimal management of ankle syndesmosis injuries. Open Access J Sports Med 2014;5:173–82.

36. Brown KW, Morrison WB, Schweitzer ME, et al. MRI findings associated with distal tibiofibular syndesmosis injury. AJR Am J Roentgenol 2004;182(1):131–6.

37. Ewalefo SO, Dombrowski M, Hirase T, et al. Management of posttraumatic ankle arthritis: literature review. Curr Rev Musculoskelet Med 2018;11(4):546–57.

38. Kramer WC, Hendricks KJ, Wang J. Pathogenetic mechanisms of posttraumatic osteoarthritis: opportunities for early intervention. Int J Clin Exp Med 2011;4: 285–98.

39. Faleiro TB, Schulz Rda S, Jambeiro JE, et al. Viscosupplementation in ankle osteoarthritis: a systematic review. Acta Ortop Bras 2016;24(1):52–4.

40. Roussignol X. Arthroscopic tibiotalar and subtalar joint arthrodesis. Orthop Traumatol Surg Res 2016;102(1 Suppl):S195–203.

41. Menz HB, Dufour AB, Casey VA, et al. Foot pain and mobility limitations in older adults: the Framingham Foot Study. J Gerontol A Biol Sci Med Sci 2013;68(10): 1281.
42. Bowes J, Buckley R. Fifth metatarsal fractures and current treatment. World J Orthop 2016;7(12):793–800.
43. Smith MS. Metatarsal fractures. In: Eiff MP, Hatch R, editors. Fracture management for primary care. 3rd edition. Philadelphia: Elsevier; 2012. p. 299–318.
44. Hossain M, Clutton J, Ridgewell M, et al. Stress fractures of the foot. Clin Sports Med 2015;34(4):769–90.
45. Goff JD, Crawford R. Diagnosis and treatment of plantar fasciitis. Am Fam Physician 2011;84(6):676–82.
46. Hsiao MY, Hung CY, Chang KV, et al. Comparative effectiveness of autologous blood-derived products, shock-wave therapy and corticosteroids for treatment of plantar fasciitis: a network meta-analysis. Rheumatology (Oxford) 2015; 54(9):1735–43.
47. Landorf KB. Plantar heel pain and plantar fasciitis. BMJ Clin Evid 2015;2015 [pii: 1111].
48. Gollwitzer H, Saxena A, DiDomenico LA, et al. Clinically relevant effectiveness of focused extracorporeal shock wave therapy in the treatment of chronic plantar fasciitis: a randomized, controlled multicenter study. J Bone Joint Surg Am 2015;97(9):701–8.
49. Mayer SW, Joyner PW, Almekinders LC, et al. Stress fractures of the foot and ankle in athletes. Sports Health 2013;6(6):481–91.
50. Mountjoy M, Sundgot-Borgen JK, Burke LM, et al. IOC consensus statement on relative energy deficiency in sport (RED-S): 2018 update. Br J Sports Med 2018;52(11):687–97.
51. Guelfi M, Pantalone A, Mirapeix RM, et al. Anatomy, pathophysiology and classification of posterior tibial tendon dysfunction. Eur Rev Med Pharmacol Sci 2017; 21(1):13–9.
52. Durrant B, Chockalingam N, Hashmi F. Posterior tibial tendon dysfunction: a review. J Am Podiatr Med Assoc 2011;101(2):176–86.

Back Injuries

James M. Daniels, MD, MPH[a],*, Cesar Arguelles, MD[a],
Christopher Gleason, MD[b], William H. Dixon, MD[a]

KEYWORDS

- Athlete • Back pain • LS spine • Spondylolysis • Spondylolisthesis • Evaluation
- Treatment • Overview

KEY POINTS

- Our definition of an athlete is a person between the ages of 14 to 65 who is active physically.
- Athletes have different demographics for back pain than the general population.
- Lumbosacral spine injury/pain is common in our country. This makes it difficult to separate the "background noise" of the whole population from the injury/pain that athletes have.
- When evaluating athletes with back pain, a broad diagnostic approach should be started so nonmusculoskeletal sources of back pain are not missed.

PREVALENCE: COMPARING APPLES WITH APPLES

If ever there was a subject in the field of musculoskeletal medicine that could use more clinically based research, it would be in the area of back pain in the athlete. There are a number of issues that make this task difficult. The first is to define what we mean by an athlete. "Athletes" can vary in age, intensity of activity, and desire for ongoing participation. A 60-year-old golfer may have different goals about treatment of his back pain than a 27-year-old carpenter who plays tournament softball in her free time. As a clinician, you may approach the evaluation of a 7-year-old soccer star brought in for evaluation after 30 days of night time back pain differently than a 22-year-old college football offensive lineman with lumbar back pain occurring 1 day after playing in a particularly hard fought game.

A second issue is that lumbar back pain is a very common problem in the general population with an estimate of 85% to 95% lifetime incidence.[1,2] One large meta-analysis estimated that the overall incidence for low back pain in athletes to be between 1% and 94%.[3]

---

[a] Department of Family and Community Medicine, Southern Illinois University School of Medicine, 612 North 11th Street, Quincy, IL 62301, USA; [b] Department of Family and Community Medicine, Southern Illinois University School of Medicine, 520 North 4th Street, Springfield, IL 62702, USA
* Corresponding author.
E-mail address: jdaniels@siumed.edu

Prim Care Clin Office Pract 47 (2020) 147–164
https://doi.org/10.1016/j.pop.2019.10.008
0095-4543/20/© 2019 Elsevier Inc. All rights reserved.

A final and a most difficult point is not simply diagnosing that the patient has low back pain; it is determining why the patient has low back pain. Most would agree that our 60-year-old golfer could probably live with an arthritic facet joint that was aggravated by golfing and weak abdominal core muscles, whereas a 7-year-old with back pain at night would need a more aggressive and different evaluation. Even though this young man plays soccer, his sport may have little to do with the etiology of his pain.

For the purposes of this article, we are going to confine our discussion to patients 14 to 65 years of age who participate in athletic activities or sports. Patients younger than 14 years of age have a higher rate of having congenital, infectious, cancerous, and inflammatory causes of their pain.[3] This group of patients is better served by another discussion about back pain in children. Patients over 65 years of age are less likely to be exposed to intense work and strain on their back as their younger counterparts. These patients most often have a different set of conditions than younger, more active athletes that we discuss here.[3]

Even when articles in the literature control for age, intensity (many studies on Olympic and National Collegiate Athletic Association athletes), and duration at presentation of symptoms (missing 3 training session in 2 weeks), there remain some obstacles to overcome. In the past, certain athletes, that is, gymnasts, soccer players, and linemen in football, were reported to have an increased incidence of back pain than other sports (basketball, nonpitchers in baseball). This difference faded when intensity of activity was controlled.[3,4] In the past many of our assumptions about sport injuries were made from data available from the National Collegiate Athletic Association, US Military, and Olympic Training Centers. When these data were analyzed further and other influences were taken into account (intensity, type of injury, return to play data), many of these differences were no longer present.

Two recent studies used meta-analysis to evaluate the groups of patients that are relevant to our discussion. The first study evaluated 1609 citations from the recent literature.[4] The second searched 6 databases (PubMed, Embase, Medline, Cochrane Library, PsysINFO, and PSYNDEX) to extract information.[3] These studies noted that the data related to various metrics (body mass index, height, range of motion, back strength) was not the same for athletes (active patients) as it was for the general population (**Table 1**). Nonathletes have an increased lifetime prevalence of low back pain

Table 1
Comparison of the demographics between athletes and control group of the general population for low back pain

	General Population	Our Population
Prevalence low back pain	+	+
Decreased lumbar flex	−	+
Hip flexor tightness	−	+
↑ Body mass index	−	+
↑ Height	+	−
Flexion/extension strength and endurance	−	+
High work load	+	U-shaped
Psych/social issues	+	Not studied

Data from Trompeter K, Fett D, Platen P. Prevalence of back pain sports: A systematic review of the literature. Sports Med. 2017;47(6):1183–1207; and Moradi V, Memari A, ShayestehFar M, et al. Low back pain in athletes is associated with general and sport specific risk factors: A comprehensive review of longitudinal studies. Rehabil Res Pract. 2015;850184:1–10.

associated with increased height of the patient while there was no increased preva-lence with a higher body mass index. Athletes, in contrast, had an increased lifetime prevalence of low back pain with a higher body mass index, but there was no associ-ation with height of the participants. In fact, basketball players had the lowest lifetime prevalence of low back pain from any group followed.[3,4]

One high quality study used a "flexaid" to measure range of motion of the lumbar spine of athletes, and it did show that decreased flexion/extension of the lumbosacral (LS) spine contributed increased risk of back pain.[3] This technique does not have wide clinical use and standards for range of motion cutoffs have not been established.[3] Hip flexor tightness and core weakness were not associated with an increased risk of low back pain in the general population, although it is in the athletic population. Workload and a history of low back pain increased the risk of low back pain in the general pop-ulation. In the nonathlete population, a history of injury is strongly correlated with future risks of low back pain, although workload results differ. In the athletic population there is a bimodal curve or a U-shaped distribution, and the patients with relatively high workloads and lower workloads have increased pain.[4]

DIAGNOSIS

When evaluating athletes with low back pain, 3 questions should be answered.

Question 1. Is the Pain Coming from the Back or Is the Pain a Symptom of Another Illness or Condition?

Several signs and symptoms are correlated with systemic causes of low back pain (**Table 2**). These are also known as red flags because they can be associated with

Table 2
List of physical examination and history points and relationship to nonmusculoskeletal causes of low back pain in the athletic population

History and Examination	General Category	Example
Fever History of urinary tract infection History of skin infection	Infection	Osteolytic Discitis Epidural abscess (neurologic defects)
	Referred pain	Pressure Pyelonephritis Pelvic inflammatory disease Endocarditis Muscle abscess Appendicitis
Worst pain 1 h in the morning Worst pain at rest	Inflammatory	Ankylosing spondylitis Reactive Inflammatory bowel associated Psoatic
Weight loss Night pain	Neoplasm	Malignant Benign Solid tumor
Other medical condition	Referral	Sickle cell Syrinx Kidney stone Tumor

Data from Hollingworth P. Back pain in children. Br J Rheumatol. 1996;35:1022–8; and Kriss VM. My aching back: a serious complaint in children. Curr Probl Diagn Radiol. 1986;16:25.

serious medical illness. A history of fever, weight loss, and/or night pain all require further investigation. A certain percentage of children with hemopoietic neoplasms present with only complaints of back or leg pain.[5,6] A further medical evaluation is useful when providing care for these patients (**Box 1**).

Along with history, causes of atypical back pain can be diagnosed with the help of a few basic laboratory tests. A complete blood count with differential, erythrocyte sedimentation rate, and C-reactive protein may help to delineate infection or hemopoietic diseases.[7] Urinalysis is also useful, although it is not very specific with identifying urinary tract infections. A lactate dehydrogenase should be ordered. If elevated, it can be associated with bone marrow conditions. The use of HLA-B27 and Lyme serology are not recommended because they have poor specificity and are prone to false-negative as well as false-positive reports.[7]

Question 2. If This Is an Issue with the Lumbosacral Spine, Is It Surgical?

Any patients with documented motor weakness should be evaluated immediately and a consult with a spine surgeon should be obtained. These patients may have unstable or progressive lesions that need urgent treatment. These lesions are not common outside of acute traumatic injuries, that is, auto accident or catastrophic athletic injury. Patients with low back pain and groin numbness or having difficulty urinating should be evaluated urgently for cauda equina syndrome. If urgent MRI is not available, urgent computed tomography scan and surgical consultation should be obtained.

There has been much written about what physical examination maneuvers are useful in evaluating athletes with LS pain. A number of physical examination techniques are well-supported by the literature (**Box 2**).[7]

The athletic population of patients differs from others by the fact that the great majority are very driven to continue participating in their sport or activity without sacrificing performance. Many athletes have musculoskeletal conditions that would resolve with rest, but these patients often do not want to stop or modify their sporting activity without some type of diagnosis and rehabilitation plan.

A more complex diagnostic evaluation should be used when evaluating athletes. To understand this evaluation process, some specific anatomy and physical examination techniques should be discussed. In this group of patients, it is very important to consider the type of trunk motion that recreates their spine pain. During evaluation, the anatomy of the LS spine should be understood and the spine is often separated into anterior and posterior compartments (**Fig. 1**). When the athlete's pain is

---

Box 1
Laboratory tests to consider ordering to aid in the evaluation of athletes with nonmusculoskeletal low back pain[a]

- Complete blood count with differential
- Erythrocyte sedimentation rate
- C-reactive protein
- Blood culture
- Urinalysis
- Complete metabolic panel – lactate dehydrogenase and uric acid

[a] HLA-B27, antinuclear antibody, Lyme serology: generally not useful.
Data from Hollingworth P. Back pain in children. Br J Rheumatol. 1996;35:1022–8; and Kriss VM. My aching back: a serious complaint in children. Curr Probl Diagn Radiol. 1986;16:25.

Box 2
Physical examination and techniques that are evidence-based in the literature for the evaluation of low back pain

Examination	Notes
L5	First toe raise, ankle dorsiflex (motor weakness, nerve tension)
S1	Ankle plantar flexion, ankle jerk (motor weakness, nerve tension)
Straight leg raise or modified slump test	Patient supine position, affected leg, hip flex 25°–30°
	Positive test – pain reproduced in leg below the knee (sensitive test)
Cross-table straight leg test	Patient supine; opposite leg, hip flex 25°–30°
	Positive test – pain reproduced in this opposite leg below the knee (specific test)
Inability to urinate	Can be side effect of medication, but sensitive test for cauda equina syndrome
Internal rotation of hip	Internal rotation of affected hip reproduces pain in groin (sensitive test for hip joint pathology)

Data from Refs.[7–9]

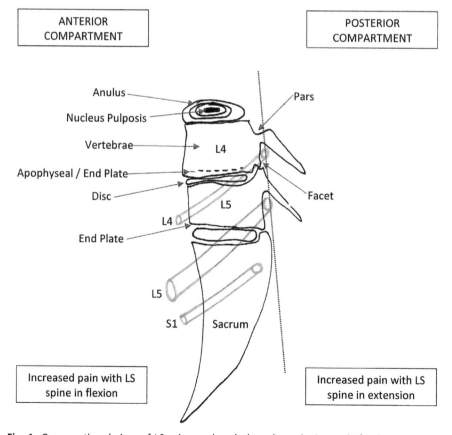

Fig. 1. Cross-sectional view of LS spine and pathology (anterior/posterior) spine.

reproduced by forward flexion of the LS spine in the absence of acute trauma and systemic causes, the following conditions should be considered.

a. *Herniated nucleus pulposus.* This condition is not that common in this group of patients. In the general population, the disc usually herniates laterally onto the existing nerve root, causing leg symptoms. This happens because the ligament flavum protects the anterior center aspect of the disc. When athletes herniate their disc, some do so anteriorly right on the dura and ventral aspect of the spinal canal. In this case, the athlete complains of low back and sacroiliac joint pain for prolonged periods of time that is aggravated by LS spine flexion. They have few or no leg symptoms. These patients usually recover in approximately 12 weeks without any procedure.

b. *Discogenic pain.* An injured disc can cause pain similar to a herniated nucleus pulposus, but is not associated with any leg pain. The main way to differentiate this condition from a herniated disc is a physical examination with MRI findings matching, that is, LS spine pain with forward flexion and normal neurologic examination despite 4 weeks of intense physical therapy while refraining from competition. The MRI often shows a high signal intensity zone in the posterior annular fibrosis.[10,11]

c. *Injury to the vertebral end plate.* This injury is difficult to separate from discogenic pain but has been described by Modic and colleagues.[12,13] Based on MRI findings, this injury is classified into 3 different types (**Fig. 2**).

d. *Apophyseal ring fracture.* This fracture can present just like a patient with disc injury. Most cases of disc injury resolve spontaneously, but nerve compression secondary to apophyseal ring fracture may not. MRI does not always differentiate between disc herniation and ring fractures. Athletes with persistent bilateral tightness of both hamstrings may have an undiagnosed apophyseal ring fracture. The exact diagnosis of an apophyseal ring fracture can be made by computed tomography; MRI can miss this entity.

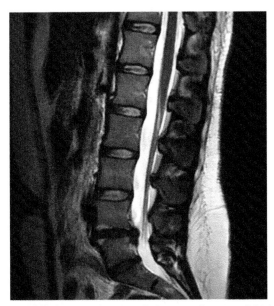

Fig. 2. This image demonstrates Modic type I lesions on the L5 and S1 levels. Observe the light color areas on the edge of each vertebrae. This type of finding is associated with central disc herniation.

When extension of the LS spine reproduces the patient's pain in the absence of acute trauma and systemic causes, the following conditions should be considered.

a. *Spondylolysis* (acute versus chronic). Acute spondylolysis is a stress fracture of the pars interarticularis when the pain is from an acute fracture. Chronic spondylolysis pain is caused by communicating synovitis of this "pseudojoint." Treatment of these 2 entities is somewhat controversial. Some authors recommend the use of MRI and use of a hard lordotic brace to treat acute spondylolysis, while using a computed tomography scan to differentiate chronic spondylolysis. A chronic lesion has no bone edema or blood. To differentiate between these 2 entities, imaging is required along with history.

b. *Facet pain.* It is rare for extension alone to cause pain in an athlete without spondylolysis. Pain with extension made worse by rotation usually is caused by facet overload, facet joint injury, facet ligament injury, or facet ligament laxity. The pain is usually from the contralateral side of the throwing arm in athletes who participate in throwing sports.

Have the patient stand straight and then have them laterally flex.

a. *Modic changes.* In patients who experience persistent pain with lateral bending that persists, an MRI short T1 inversion recovery image may show type I Modic changes, bone bruising (discussed elsewhere in this article). This finding is often overlooked and may be of use for athletes, who play sports requiring a significant amount of truncal rotation such as golf, gymnastics, and diving, with persistent pain despite adequate treatment.

Physical examination techniques are helpful in this particular population (**Fig. 3**). These tests lose their usefulness in other patient populations. First, observe the patient from the side (see **Fig. 3**A) to evaluate their sagittal balance. In other words, look for lordosis of C-spine, kyphosis of T-spine, and lordosis of the LS spine. The examiner should be able to drop a plumb bob from the patient's ear and the line would intersect to the pelvis laterally. Observe the patient in formal flexion (see **Fig. 3**B), then extension (see **Fig. 3**C). Observe if either maneuver accentuates pain. Then have the patient move side to side (see **Fig. 3**D, E). If pain is present, consider Modic changes or vertebral bruising (see **Fig. 2**). The concept of sagittal balance can help to explain why other parts of the spine can affect the LS spine.[14,15]

If none of these positions reproduce the patient's pain, stress maneuvers can be used to help reproduce the patient's pain (**Fig. 4**). The dead cockroach position (see **Fig. 4**A) evaluates the patient's ability to hold their arms and legs out in space without pain. The side plank (see **Fig. 4**B) and flying lateral plank (see **Fig. 4**C) on each side of the patient demonstrates core strength, and super(wo)man positions (see **Fig. 4**D, E) evaluate core strength in extension. Using a 2-step evaluation process allows the examiner to (a) evaluate the patient's ability to assume a neutral spine position, and (b) the second set evaluates the strength and endurance of the LS spine. We use the supine patient's test to evaluate the patient's ability to control the musculature in the LS spine along with evaluating the patient's strength. The patient is placed in a supine position with knee flexed 45° to 60° (**Fig. 5**A). Then the examiner places their hand at the junction of the LS spine and sacrum (**Fig. 5**B). The patient is asked to raise and then push back against the examiner's hand. The ability and force are evaluated. This test is very useful when diagnosing back pain, but even more useful evaluating the ability of the patient to hold neutral spine and the endurance of the core musculature.

A few tests are also useful not only in diagnosing but treating athletes with low back pain. A standard straight leg test may not demonstrate leg pain in this population. The

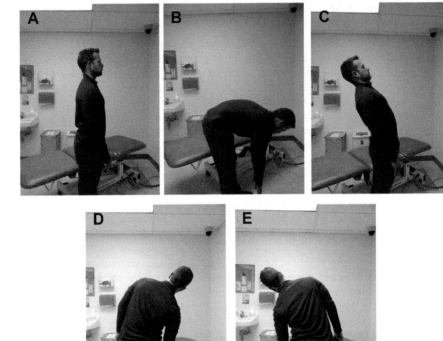

Fig. 3. Initial maneuvers to evaluate range of motion and posture of athletes with low back pain. (*A*) Lateral standing position to observe the patient's sagittal balance. (*B*) Forward flexion. (*C*) Back extension. (*D*, *E*) Lateral flexion, both directions.

slump test (**Fig. 6**) has the patient flex their C-spine and flexes the hip to 90° while completely extending their knee. This maneuver puts extra traction on the cord and may allow for a more sensitive straight leg test for this population.[14]

After metabolic and mechanical causes of low back pain are evaluated and red flags have been investigated, the third clinical question should be considered.

PROGNOSIS
Question 3. Why Is This Athlete Not Improving with Rest?

There has been a moderate amount of investigation into this question. A number of questions have been designed specifically for athletes to rule out psychological or stress factors that could be interfering with recovery in athletes with LS spine injuries. One version REST-Q-Basic failed to correlate stress and back pain in competitive athletes.[16] Psychosocial Risk Stratification Index, Risk Prevention Index and receiver operating characteristics demonstrated significantly lower psychosocial risk profiles and prognostic risks in athletes as compared with nonathletes.[17] So there is evidence that despite having some risk factors (challenging schedules, overly demanding coach, parents, etc) for developing psychological symptoms, athletes seem to have a decreased risk for stress-related conditions than their peers who do not view themselves as athletes. With that said, there were some nonathletic risk factors associated

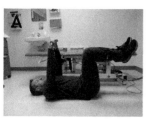
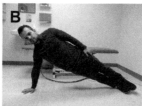
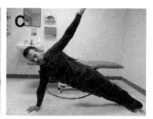
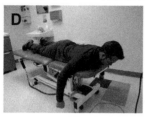
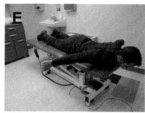

Fig. 4. These maneuvers can be used during a physical examination to evaluate an athlete's strength and endurance. These same maneuvers can be given as home exercises. The maneuvers should only be used if the patient is relatively pain free and can easily demonstrate the maneuvers described. (*A*) The cockroach position strengthens hip and core muscles. (*B*) The side plank fires core and lower extremity muscles and requires coordination. (*C*) The flying lateral plank adds coordination of upper extremity to maneuver. (*D, E*) The super(wo)man fires extensor muscles in prone position and abduction.

with back pain in adolescent athletes: late bed time, short sleeping time, and excessive video gaming.[18]

Athletes are a part of the general population and can become depressed or anxious. Many adolescents identify with a sport or activity on a number of levels. A good example is an athlete may say. "I am a football player" or "I am a cheerleader" when asked to describe themselves. This activity plays a key role in the athlete's self-identity structure. In addition, the athletes' social activities may revolve around

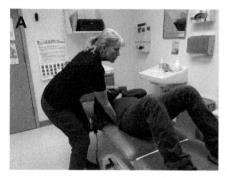
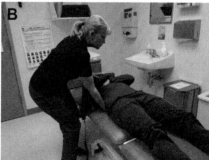

Fig. 5. Specific maneuvers to evaluate athletes with low back pain. (*A*) Supine neutral spine test. The athlete is supine with knees bent about 45°. Examiner places hand at the juncture of spine and sacrum, then asks the patient to "push against my hand." This evaluates ability to flex the LS spine. (A blood pressure cuff pumped to 40 mm can be substituted for hand and amount of rise can be recorded instead of using hand.) Then ask the patient to "arch away" from hand. This measures the ability of the athlete to extend the LS spine. (*B*) The whole process can be repeated with athlete's knees completely extended (makes the test more difficult).

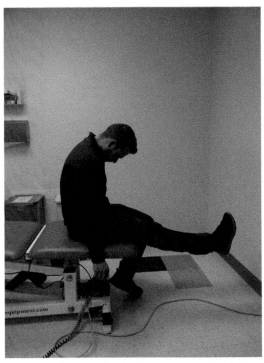

Fig. 6. Slump test for the evaluation of radicular symptoms in athletes C-spine flexed, hip flexed at 90°, knee extended. The test is positive if it reproduces the patient's pain below the tested knee.

their teammates. If an athlete is totally away from their sport or teammate, they may become anxious or depressed. If they believe for some reason that they may not be able to return to their previous level of play, they may develop significant mental health issues. Additionally, exercise itself is commonly used as a stress reducer. If an athlete is injured and away from the sport for as little as a week, they may become stressed and anxious.[16,17,19] The Patient Health Questionnaire-2 is an easy to administer survey tool that can be used when evaluating athletes with back injuries or pain (**Fig. 7**). It is composed of 2 questions: (1) Do you have little interest or pleasure in doing things? and (2) Are you feeling down, depressed, or hopeless? If either one of these answers are positive or if the athlete has a hard time answering them, a counselor should be consulted if the clinician is either uncomfortable or has no prior training in cognitive–behavioral therapy. There is less and less controversy now that psychosocial issues can play a bias role in the delay of recovery of patients with back pain.[16,17,19]

CLINICAL MANAGEMENT

The general approach to an athlete with LS pain is outlined in **Tables 1** and **2** and **Boxes 1** and **2**. This evaluation included evaluating patient demographics, history, physical examination, and differential diagnosis based on the patient's symptoms and pain. Mechanical issues of the spine can be classified into anterior and posterior anatomic structures and important imaging findings (see **Figs. 1** and **2**).

A

The Patient Health Questionnaire-2 (PHQ-2)

Patient Name _____ Date of Visit _____

Over the past 2 weeks, how often have you been bothered by any of the following problems?	Not At all	Several Days	More Than Half the Days	Nearly Every Day
1. Little interest or pleasure in doing things	0	1	2	3
2. Feeling down, depressed or hopeless	0	1	2	3

B

asQ Ask Suicide-Screening Questions

NIMH TOOLKIT

Suicide Risk **Screening Tool**

Ask the patient:

1. In the past few weeks, have you wished you were dead? ○ Yes ○ No

2. In the past few weeks, have you felt that you or your family would be better off if you were dead? ○ Yes ○ No

3. In the past week, have you been having thoughts about killing yourself? ○ Yes ○ No

4. Have you ever tried to kill yourself? ○ Yes ○ No

   If yes, how? _____

   _____

   When? _____

   _____

If the patient answers Yes to any of the above, ask the following acuity question:

5. Are you having thoughts of killing yourself right now? ○ Yes ○ No

   If yes, please describe: _____

Next steps:

- If patient answers "No" to all questions 1 through 4, screening is complete (not necessary to ask question #5). No intervention is necessary (*Note: Clinical judgment can always override a negative screen).
- If patient answers "Yes" to any of questions 1 through 4, or refuses to answer, they are considered a positive screen. Ask question #5 to assess acuity:
  - □ "Yes" to question #5 = acute positive screen (imminent risk identified)
    - **Patient requires a STAT safety/full mental health evaluation.** Patient cannot leave until evaluated for safety.
    - Keep patient in sight. Remove all dangerous objects from room. Alert physician or clinician responsible for patient's care.
  - □ "No" to question #5 = non-acute positive screen (potential risk identified)
    - **Patient requires a brief suicide safety assessment to determine if a full mental health evaluation is needed.** Patient cannot leave until evaluated for safety.
    - Alert physician or clinician responsible for patient's care.

Provide resources to all patients

- 24/7 National Suicide Prevention Lifeline 1-800-273-TALK (8255) En Español: 1-888-628-9454
- 24/7 Crisis Text Line: Text "HOME" to 741-741

asQ Suicide Risk Screening Toolkit NATIONAL INSTITUTE OF MENTAL HEALTH (NIMH) 4/13/2017

Fig. 7. Psychosocial tools to rule out depression and/or risk of suicide. (*A*) Patient Health Questionnaire-2 (Developed by Drs. R.L. Spitzer, J.B. Williams, K. Kroenke and colleagues with an educational grant from Pfizer, Inc. No permission required to reproduce, translate, display or distribute.). (*B*) The asQ Suicide Risk Screening Tool. (*From* National Institute of Mental Health. asQ suicide risk screening tool. Available at: https://www.nimh.nih.gov/research/research-conducted-at-nimh/asq-toolkit-materials/asq-tool/screening-tool_155867.pdf.)

The next step in management after making a diagnosis can be subdivided into patients with (a) red flags—signs or symptoms of serious medical conditions that requires urgent treatment (**Box 3**), (b) consultation and/or hospitalization needed, (c) patients with symptoms for less than 2 weeks in duration who do not seem to have emergent medical conditions, and (d) patients with symptoms for more than 2 weeks in duration who do not seem to have an emergent condition.

Box 3
Reasons for urgent consult or hospitalization in athletes with low back pain

- Sepsis suspected
- Diagnosis of solid tumor or hemopoietic disease
- Discitis or osteomyelitis suspected
- History of trauma with unstable fracture
- Patients with motor weakness
- Vertebral fractures
- Progression of spondylolisthesis
- Scheuermann kyphosis
- Scoliosis of 20° or more when patient still has open apophysis

Data from McGhee JL, Burks FN, Scheckels JL, et al. Identifying children with chronic arthritis based on chief complaints: absence of predictive value for musculoskeletal pain as an indicator of rheumatic disease in children. Pediatrics. 2002;110:354–9; and Miller R, Beck NA, Sampson NR, et al. Imaging modalities for low back pain in children: a review of spondylolysis and undiagnosed mechanical back pain. J Pediatr Orthop. 2013;33:282–8.

Most patients with pain of 2 weeks duration or less (70%–90%) improve regardless of treatment.[20–22] The activities that aggravate their back symptoms should be avoided and patients should not be placed on strict bedrest (unless history of trauma and awaiting imaging).[23] A reasonable treatment plan would be to allow school and work, but avoid activities that specifically aggravate the condition (see **Fig. 1**). Some type of physical activity should be encouraged but full participation in sports may not be possible if it involves contact or aggravates condition. A short course of nonsteroidal anti-inflammatory drugs (NSAIDs) has been found to be superior in relieving patient's pain when compared with acetaminophen.[24] It should be explained to the patients that NSAIDs are used strictly for pain reduction. They do not decrease inflammation or make tissues heal any faster. Additionally, patients with suspected or proven gastrointestinal ulcers or kidney disease should not use this medications and patients should be made aware of the possible associated between the use of NSAID and sustaining an acute myocardial infarction.[25,26]

The addition of cyclobenzaprine is reasonable treatment option. When taken at night it aids in sleep. It is a stereoisomer of amitriptyline so it increases rapid eye movement sleep as opposed to other sleeping aids that decrease rapid eye movement sleep.[27,28] Although ice has not proven to stop inflammation or effect circulation to the affected muscles, it does have some analgesic effect.[29] The use of opioids and tramadol should be reserved for fractures, trauma or other severe injury. The side effects of overprescribing these medications are well known in primary care medicine today. Systemic steroids should not be used as they not only do not help alleviate back pain and they can cause significant harm.[27,28]

A number of studies evaluated modalities and treatments for patients with back pain (**Table 3**). In summary, the evidence-based treatment of low back pain (after a proper workup, as described elsewhere in this article) in athletes with symptoms less than 2 weeks in duration include keeping the patient active but modify their activities that aggravate the condition, encourage use of topical creams, NSAIDs over acetaminophen, ice/heat, and, if they wish, spinal manipulation.

Table 3
A list of various integrative modalities/treatment for athletes with low back pain

Modality or Treatment	Effectiveness
Topical creams	Moderate evidence helps with pain[30]
Heat	Short term, should not lay on active heat generator for long periods of time, that is, going to sleep with heating pad on back; hot shower to limber up (E30)
Massage	No evidence it helps, but patient enjoy it[31]
Acupuncture	Inconsistent outcomes but safe[32]
Spinal manipulation	Moderate evidence it helped[33]
Physical therapy	Has moderate evidence it helped[34,35]
Ice	Does not stop inflammation, but may help with pain
Muscle energy technique	No evidence it helps[36]
Traction	With or without radiculopathy – it helps[37]
Lumbar supports	Does not help; if overused, it could cause harm[38]
Change mattress	Unless mattress has a large "sag" in the middle, and so on, no type is better than the other

Those athletes with pain lasting more than 2 weeks can undergo the same initial treatment but should be evaluated for specific movements that aggravate their condition (see **Fig. 3**). If the proper laboratory tests and spinal radiographs have not been obtained, they should be ordered. Consultation with a physical therapist, qualified certified athletic trainer, or chiropractor should be considered after all nonmechanical causes have been ruled out. Patients should be followed up within 2 weeks of being evaluated. If treatment helped and/or a specific diagnosis and treatment plan are made, the patient should be followed up appropriately. If the athlete is no better, develops worsening symptoms, or no obvious diagnosis is present, the patient can be referred to a spinal specialist. In real-world case scenarios, it is often not possible to get a patient without a surgical diagnosis or an emergent problem in to be evaluated. Many clinicians will at that point order advanced imaging. These authors would argue that a phone call to the consultant should be made before ordering studies for the following reasons. (1) The consultant may make special arrangements to see the patient because you took time to call him or her. (2) The consultant may have other ideas or recommendations that they can give you over the phone. (3) The proper diagnostic test can be ordered.

CONTROVERSIES

Various imaging techniques that can be used to help diagnose athletes with back pain and the pros/cons associated with their use are available (**Table 4**).

Many health care providers contend that the key to prevent reoccurring back pain in athletes with chronic back pain with no surgical or metabolic diagnosis is rehabilitation of core or abdominal and hip muscles.[42,43] As the athlete recovers from an injury of the LS spine, there are many professionals who advocate the introduction of core exercises to strengthen abdominal and hip muscles (see **Fig. 4**).[42] Although some clinicians argue that there is no good way to measure or identify improvement in muscle strength of the core,[44] others argue and show evidence that demonstration of muscle strength improvement is not necessary. There is evidence that a trunk stabilizing program does not allow athletes to return to strenuous activity sooner, but it may help to prevent recurrence of

Table 4
Imaging techniques and their pros and cons in athletes with low back pain

Image	Pros	Cons
AP, lateral and oblique radiographs of the LS spine	Standard practice for years Able to pick up spondylolysis later in its course Grade spondylolisthesis Easy to obtain	Lots of radiation Can now pick up spondylolysis earlier with other imaging modalities Athlete is laying in supine position Cannot access spinal curves
Standing Lateral and AP radiographs of the LS spine	Much less radiation Better way to access natural curve in LS spine	
MRI without access	Hands down best test when patient has abnormal neurologic examination Radicular symptoms Known or suspected malignancy Suspected cord compression Useful in detecting discitis Spinal cord inflammation SI inflammation	Expensive Sometimes difficult to schedule Patient has to be confined in supine position for a long period of time Can have difficulty differentiating "hot spots"
MRI with contrast	Ability to differentiate old scar tissue from new lesions	–
Bone scan	Cheap Easy to order Very sensitive in detecting early spondylolysis vs just bone reaction Negative scan virtually negates spondylolysis Can differentiate between old fracture and new Higher correlation with spondylolysis than MRI	Radiation MRI better for infection, inflammation Evaluation neurologic structure
SPCT/CT CT only done if bone scan hot	Easy to order Relatively cheap Only thin area 1 level CT done not complete CT Is about equivalent of old "oblique views" in regard to radiation Don't have to fit in gantry Very helpful with return to play decisions	
CT	Cheap Available No worries with gantries Good at bone resolution	Radiation Poor soft tissue resolution compared with MRI

Abbreviations: AP, anteroposterior; CT, computed tomography; MRI, magnetic resonance imaging; SI, sacroiliac.
Data from Refs.[15,39–41]

injuries that prevent the athlete from competing.[42,43,45,46] These studies were not long term, with the studies spanning months, not years.

When treating athletes with spondylolysis and spondylolisthesis, a short review of this condition is helpful. There are 5 types of spondylolysis and **Table 5** describes them. Type I spondylolisthesis is congenital. There is rounding of the first sacral vertebra. Type II is from a stress fracture of the pars articularis. Type III is caused from degenerative changes in the facets and is associated with older patients. Types IV and V are caused by trauma or bone disorder. Type II or isthmic spondylolisthesis is the most common type in athletes and type I has the highest risk of progression.[47]

Athletes with type II spondylolysis were commonly treated with a rigid kyphotic back brace that was worn 23 hours a day. These were lightweight and custom made for each athlete. There were some compliance issues with these boards and other researchers believed it was more appropriate to place the athlete in a lordotic brace to assist in healing by pressing the 2 sides of the fracture together. These athletes had similar outcomes, which led another group to treat these patients with no brace or a soft type brace. It was found that removing the athlete from play for 1 season (3–4 months) would allow these lesions to heal and isometric exercises were used to help strengthen core abdominal muscles as opposed to the 23-hour use of a brace that would weaken those same muscles.[41]

Many physicians continue to forego the brace for certain athletes, that is, type II spondylolysis (little or no spondylolysis) respond by avoidance of aggravating activities, an agreement with the health care provider, parent and/or coach to rest, and no motor defects.[41]

Table 5
Wiltse classification of spondylolisthesis

Type	Description	Illustration
I	Congenital Due rounding of the superior ventral surface on the first sacral vertebra, most common type to slip	
II	Most common in young athlete, caused by stress fracture of the pars articularis	
III	No fracture or problem with pars Usually from overload of facets Causing overload of the facet and development of arthritis Facets do not fit together well and ligaments are stretched	
IV and V	Caused from trauma or generalized bone disease, respectively	

Data from Moore D. Adult isthmic spondylolisthesis. Available at: https://www.orthobullets.com/spine/2038/adult-isthmic-spondylolisthesis. Accessed March 31, 2019.

Older athletes with herniated discs that did not respond to 90 days of conservative therapy, including the use of epidural steroid treatment, or those who could or would not be able to abstain from aggravating activities that long have opted to undergo a percutaneous endoscopic dissection performed with or without laser ablation. This type of surgery can be performed under local anesthesia using an 8-mm skin incision with minimal or no injury to the lumbar spine musculature.[48] Many of these athletes return to play in as little as 6 weeks for noncontact sports and 8 weeks for contact sports. More traditional surgery such as microendoscopic discectomy remove the herniated disc material through the interlaminar space (more ligaments cut) compared with the percutaneous endoscopic dissection, which removes the disc through the intervertebral foramen.[49] Athletes undergoing the percutaneous endoscopic dissection procedure have an increased risk of certain complications, including damage to the nerve root during canula insertion and development of high intercranial and epidural pressures. Athletes may have a tendency to take on this increased risk to return to sport early. Insurance companies may favor these procedures because of the ability to perform then as an outpatient in stepdown operating theaters. The treating physician should mind the old prose, "It's all about the archer, not the arrow" when discussing this with the patient. The most experienced surgeon using the best, safest procedure that they are familiar with should take precedence over a pathway that allows a return to activity a few months earlier by using a new untested procedure.

DISCLOSURE

The authors have nothing to disclose.

REFERENCES

1. Jones T, Kumar S. Physical ergonomics in low-back pain prevention. J Occup Rehabil 2001;11(4):309–19.
2. Burton AK. How to prevent low back pain. Best Pract Res Clin Rheumatol 2005; 19:541–55.
3. Trompeter K, Fett D, Platen P. Prevalence of back pain sports: a systematic review of the literature. Sports Med 2017;47(6):1183–207.
4. Moradi V, Memari A, ShayestehFar M, et al. Low back pain in athletes is associated with general and sport specific risk factors: a comprehensive review of longitudinal studies. Rehabil Res Pract 2015;850184:1–10.
5. Hollingworth P. Back pain in children. Br J Rheumatol 1996;35:1022–8.
6. Kriss VM. My aching back: a serious complaint in children. Curr Probl Diagn Radiol 1986;16:25.
7. McGhee JL, Burks FN, Scheckels JL, et al. Identifying children with chronic arthritis based on chief complaints: absence of predictive value for musculoskeletal pain as an indicator of rheumatic disease in children. Pediatrics 2002;110: 354–9.
8. Cleland J, Koppenhaver S. Netter's orthopaedic clinical examination. Yardley (PA): Saunders; 2005. p. 201–36 [Chapter 6].
9. Miller R, Beck NA, Sampson NR, et al. Imaging modalities for low back pain in children: a review of spondylolysis and undiagnosed mechanical back pain. J Pediatr Orthop 2013;33:282–8.
10. Sairyo K, Nagamachi A. State-of-the-art management of low back pain in athletes: instructional lecture. J Orthop Sci 2016;21:263–72.
11. Aprill C, Bogduc N. High-intensity zone: a diagnostic sign of painful lumbar disc on magnetic resonance imaging. Br J Radiol 1992;65:361–9.

12. Modic MT, Steinberg PM, Ross JS, et al. Degenerative disk disease: assessment of changes in vertebral body marrow with MR imaging. Radiology 1988;166: 193–9.

13. Modic MT, Masaryk TJ, Ross JS, et al. Imaging of degenerative disk disease. Radiology 1988;168:177–86.

14. Kim JM, Freitag P. Lumbosacral spine. In: Daniels JM, editor. Common musculo-skeletal problems: a handbook. 2nd edition. (Switzerland): Springer; 2015. p. 65–75.

15. Matesan M, Behnia F, Bermo M, et al. SPECT/CT bone scintigraphy to evaluate low back pain in young athletes: common and uncommon etiologies. J Orthop Surg Res 2016. https://doi.org/10.1186/s13018-016-0402-1.

16. Heidari J, Belz J, Hasenbring M, et al. Full title: examining the presence of back pain in competitive athletes: a focus on stress and recovery. J Sport Rehabil 2017;15:1–26.

17. Wippert PM, Puschmann AK, Arampatzis A, et al. Diagnosis of psychosocial risk factors in prevention of low back pain in athletes (MiSpEx). BMJ Open Sport Exerc Med 2017;3(1):e000295.

18. Yabe Y, Hagiwara Y, Sekiguchi T, et al. Late bedtimes, short sleeping time, and longtime video-game playing are associated with low back pain in school-aged athletes. Eur Spine J 2018;27(5):1112–8.

19. Hasenbring MI, Levenig C, Hallner D, et al. Psychosocial risk factors for chronic back pain in the general population and in competitive sports: from theory to clinical screening: a review from the MiSpEx network. 2018. Available at: https://www.ncbi.nlm.nih.gov/pubmed/29946960. Accessed July 15, 2018.

20. Deyo RA, Weinstein JN. Low back pain. N Engl J Med 2001;344:363–70.

21. Coste J, Delecoeuillerie G, Cohen de Lara A, et al. Clinical course and prognostic factors in acute low back pain: an inception cohort study in primary care practice. BMJ 1994;308:577.

22. Cherkin DC, Deyo RA, Street JH, et al. Predicting poor outcomes for back pain seen in primary care using patients' own criteria. Spine (Phila Pa 1976) 1996; 21:2900.

23. Qaseem A, Wilt TJ, McLean RM, et al. Noninvasive treatments for acute, subacute, and chronic low back pain: a clinical practice guideline from the American College of Physicians. Ann Intern Med 2017;166:514.

24. Saragiotto BT, Machado GC, Ferreira ML, et al. Paracetamol for low back pain. Cochrane Database Syst Rev 2016;(6):CD012230.

25. Agency for Healthcare Research and Quality (AHRQ). Noninvasive treatments for low back pain. AHRQ Publication No. 16-EHC004-EF. 2016. Available at: https://effectivehealthcare.ahrq.gov/ehc/products/553/2178/back-pain-treatment-report-160229.pdf. Accessed on March 11, 2016.

26. Machado GC, Maher CG, Ferreira PH, et al. Non-steroidal anti-inflammatory drugs for spinal pain: a systematic review and meta-analysis. Ann Rheum Dis 2017;76(7):1269–78.

27. Beebe FA, Barkin RL, Barkin S. A clinical and pharmacologic review of skeletal muscle relaxants for musculoskeletal conditions. Am J Ther 2005;12:151.

28. Chou R, Peterson K, Helfand M. Comparative efficacy and safety of skeletal muscle relaxants for spasticity and musculoskeletal conditions: a systematic review. J Pain Symptom Manage 2004;28:140.

29. French SD, Cameron M, Walker BF, et al. Superficial heat or cold for low back pain. Cochrane Database Syst Rev 2006;(1):CD004750.

30. Abdel Shaheed C, Maher CG, Williams KA, et al. Interventions available over the counter and advice for acute low back pain: systematic review and meta-analysis. J Pain 2014;15:2.
31. Furlan AD, Giraldo M, Baskwill A, et al. Massage for low-back pain. Cochrane Database Syst Rev 2015;(4):CD001929.
32. Faas A. Exercises: which ones are worth trying, for which patients, and when? Spine (Phila Pa 1976) 1996;21:2874.
33. Paige NM, Miake-Lye IM, Booth MS, et al. Association of spinal manipulative therapy with clinical benefit and harm for acute low back pain: systematic review and meta-analysis. JAMA 2017;317:1451.
34. Brennan GP, Fritz JM, Hunter SJ, et al. Identifying subgroups of patients with acute/subacute "nonspecific" low back pain: results of a randomized clinical trial. Spine (Phila Pa 1976) 2006;31:623.
35. Fritz JM, Delitto A, Erhard RE. Comparison of classification-based physical therapy with therapy based on clinical practice guidelines for patients with acute low back pain: a randomized clinical trial. Spine (Phila Pa 1976) 2003;28:1363.
36. Franke H, Fryer G, Ostelo RW, et al. Muscle energy technique for non-specific low-back pain. Cochrane Database Syst Rev 2015;(2):CD009852.
37. Wegner I, Widyahening IS, van Tulder MW, et al. Traction for low-back pain with or without sciatica. Cochrane Database Syst Rev 2013;(8):CD003010.
38. van Duijvenbode IC, Jellema P, van Poppel MN, et al. Lumbar supports for prevention and treatment of low back pain. Cochrane Database Syst Rev 2008;(2):CD001823.
39. Dizdarevic I, Bishop M, Sgromolo N, et al. Approach to the pediatric athlete with back pain: more than just the pars. Phys Sportsmed 2015;43(4):421–31.
40. DeLuigi AJ. Low back pain in the adolescent athlete. Phys Med Rehabil Clin N Am 2014;25(4):763–88.
41. Daniels JM, Pontius G, El-Amin S, et al. Evaluation of low back pain in the athlete. Sportshealth 2011;3(4):336–45.
42. Abdelraouf OR, Abdel-Aziem AA. The relationship between core endurance and back dysfunction in collegiate male athletes with and without nonspecific low back pain. Int J Sports Phys Ther 2016;11(3):337–44.
43. Butowicz CM, Ebaugh DD, Noehren B, et al. Validation of two clinical measures of core stability. Int J Phys Ther 2016;11(1):15–23.
44. Friedrich J, Brakke R, Akuthota V, et al. Reliability and practicality of the core score: four dynamic core stability tests performed in a physician office setting. Clin J Sport Med 2017;27(4):409–14.
45. Mueller S, Stoll J, Mueller J, et al. Trunk muscle activity during drop jump performance in adolescent athletes with back pain. Front Physiol 2017;8:274.
46. Moore D. Adult Isthmic Spondylolisthesis. In: OrthoBullets. 2019. Available at: https://www.orthobullets.com/spine/2038/adult-isthmic-spondylolisthesis. Accessed March 31, 2019.
47. Jeffries LJ, Milanese SF, Grimmer-Somers KA. Epidemiology of adolescent spinal pain: a systematic overview of the research literature. Spine (Phila Pa 1976) 2007; 32:2630.
48. Sairyo K, Egawa H, Matsuura T, et al. A state of the art: transforaminal approach for percutaneous endoscopic lumbar discectomy under local anesthesia. J Med Invest 2014;61:327–32.
49. Sairyo K, Matsuura T, Higashino K, et al. Surgery related complications in percutaneous endoscopic lumbar discectomy under local anesthesia. J Med Invest 2014;61:264–9.

Neck Injuries

Benjamin Oshlag, MD[a],*, Tracy Ray, MD[b], Benjamin Boswell, DO[c]

KEYWORDS

- Neck injuries • Cervical spine • Spinal cord injury • Spinal immobilization
- Cervical collar • Sports medicine

KEY POINTS

- Neck injuries are relatively uncommon and usually self-limited, so that a full recovery can be expected.
- Catastrophic injury patterns for cervical spine injuries are often related to direct axial load trauma with a slightly forward-flexed neck, in which the normal lordotic curve is lost.
- Cervical spine imaging should begin with radiographs or computed tomography. When indicated, MRI should be used to evaluate for ligamentous, muscle, and spinal cord involvement.
- Routine cervical spine immobilization in a hard cervical collar may provide more harm than benefit in neck injuries, and a more individualized approach may be more reasonable.
- Return to play from neck injuries varies based on severity of injury, but athletes should be able to demonstrate normal strength and pain-free range of motion before they are cleared for full activity.

INTRODUCTION/BACKGROUND
Spinal Cord Injury Epidemiology

An estimated 10,000 to 11,000 spinal cord injuries (SCIs) occur each year in the United States, and approximately 10% of spinal cord injuries in the United States are related directly or indirectly to athletic events.[1] The spectrum of SCI ranges from minor and temporary "burners" or "stingers," to severe but nonpermanent fractures and impingements, to permanently disabling spinal damage, and even to fatalities. Realistically, neck injuries are relatively uncommon and usually self-limited so that a full recovery can be expected.[2] However, because of their potential to cause permanent damage to the spinal cord and even death, neck injuries have come to represent one of the most feared injuries in sports.[2,3]

---

[a] Department of Emergency Medicine, Icahn School of Medicine at Mount Sinai, Mount Sinai Beth Israel Hospital, First Ave at 16th St, New York, NY 10003, USA; [b] Duke Sports Medicine, Duke University, 3475 Erwin Rd, Durham, NC 27705, USA; [c] Dvision of Sports Medicine, Primary Care Sports Medicine, Department of Orthopedic Surgery, Department of Emergency Medicine, Case Western Reserve University School of Medicine, University Hospitals Cleveland, 11100 Euclid Avenue, Cleveland, OH 44106, USA
* Corresponding author.
E-mail address: boshlag@gmail.com

Prim Care Clin Office Pract 47 (2020) 165–176
https://doi.org/10.1016/j.pop.2019.10.009
0095-4543/20/© 2019 Elsevier Inc. All rights reserved.
primarycare.theclinics.com

Injury patterns in cervical spine injuries are seen across a wide range of sports. Sports-related cervical spine injuries are most common in athletes 30 years old or younger, with more than half occurring in those younger than 18.[1] The most common sports associated with injuries varies by region. Ice hockey injuries are more common in Canada, whereas rugby injuries are more common in Europe, South Africa, and Australia.[2]

Football notoriously contributes the highest numbers per year of head and neck injuries because of the high numbers of participants and the repetitive contact style of play.[4] Cervical spine injuries occur in roughly 10% to 15% of all football players, with the highest percentages in athletes who play defensive positions.[5] Although football is the leading cause of cervical sprains in the United States, cycling is associated with more cervical fractures in men, and horseback riding in women.[1]

Compared with female individuals, incidence of cervical spine injuries in male individuals was 1.7 times greater for neck sprains and 3.6 times greater for fractures.[1] Many other sports have proportionally high risk for SCIs as well. These range from contact sports like hockey, wrestling, and lacrosse to nonorganized sports like diving, surfing, and skiing and high-energy sports like gymnastics, cycling, and horseback riding.[1,3–5]

History

As awareness has grown of the long-term effects of head and spine injuries in all sports, there have been endeavors to protect athletes through rule changes, advanced equipment, improved medical care at athletic events, new styles of coaching, and updated practice strategies.[6] In 1976, the National Collegiate Athletic Association (NCAA) banned the practice of "spearing," a tackling technique that involves lowering the head to use the crown of the helmet as the initial point of contact, in collegiate football.[1,4,6] Over the following decades, the rate of cervical spine injuries fell by 70%, and cases of traumatic quadriplegia in US football decreased by 82%.[1,3]

There are still many cases each year of SCI during sporting events, and tracking of these injuries is largely considered to be inadequate.[5,6] Experts continue to debate standards for field-side medical action and return-to-play guidelines, a conflict that is polarizing because of the seriousness of SCI.[3] The general attitude of fear surrounding SCI in recent years has led medical professionals to use extreme caution and a rule-of-thumb approach when dealing with acute neck injuries during sporting events.[3,5,7,8] If there is any suspicion that an athlete has an SCI, the traditional practice has been to err on the side of caution and immediately immobilize the neck and spine using a "boarding" technique; however, as outlined later in this article, more recent studies indicate a need to possibly reconsider this approach.

ANATOMY OF THE CERVICAL SPINE
Overview

The cervical spine is the uppermost segment of the spinal column. It contains 7 cervical vertebrae, C1 to C7. The spinal cord passes through the center of the cervical vertebrae by way of the spinal canal, with 8 nerve roots that exit from between each vertebra. Both static and dynamic stabilizers maintain the structural integrity of the cervical spine, including bones, cartilage, ligaments, muscles, and tendons. They form a complex infrastructure, both strong and flexible, that upholds the alignment of the cervical spine, allows for a wide range of motion, and functionally dissipates and absorbs the impact of external forces to the head and neck.

Upper Cervical Spine: Atlas and Axis

The first cervical vertebra (C1) is the atlas. Unlike the normal vertebral body shape of the other spinal segments, the atlas is a ringlike structure that articulates with the occipital bone at the base of the skull, at the atlanto-occipital joint.[8] This synovial joint is composed of 2 articular capsules, 2 membranes, and 2 ligaments.[8] It connects the superior articular facets of the atlas to the occipital condyles, creating a flexible structure that allows for approximately 50% of all cervical flexion and extension, earning it the nickname of the "yes" joint.[5]

The second cervical vertebra (C2) is the axis. The axis has a typical vertebral body, but is distinguished by an upward, fingerlike projection known as the dens, or the odontoid process.[9] The odontoid process serves as a pivot point around which the ring-shaped axis rotates. The axis articulates with the atlas at the atlantoaxial joint, where the anterior arch of the atlas meets the dens.[7,8] This complex joint holds C1 and C2 together, and is responsible for the high level of mobility and rotation in the neck.[8] Two alar ligaments extend from the odontoid process to the inner border of the occipital condyles, restricting rotation in the joint.[4] The odontoid process is also attached centrally to the occipital bone at the anterior foramen magnum by the apical ligament.[4] Another stabilizing structure for C1 and C2 is the transverse atlantal ligament, which, together with the superior and inferior longitudinal bands, forms a thick, strong "cross bar" through the ring of the atlas, holding the dens securely against the anterior arch.[4,7] Lateral joint capsules contribute to the strength of the joint as well.[4] The atlantoaxial joint accounts for approximately 50% of all cervical rotation, and has been aptly called the "no" joint.[5]

Lower Cervical Spine

Although C1 and C2 and the joints between them make up the upper segment of the cervical spine, the lower segment includes C3 through C7 and ends at T1.[5,7–9] The bony structure of these vertebrae is relatively consistent: oval vertebral bodies with large triangular foramina through their transverse processes and a spinal canal that is less spacious than it is in the upper cervical spine.[4,7] C7 has a notably longer, more prominent spinous process that is often used as a palpable reference for locating the end of the cervical spine. The 45-degree angle of the facet joints of C3 to C7 allows for cervical flexion and extension while limiting axial rotation.[4] Motion in this part of the neck is coupled so that axial rotation occurs with lateral bending.[4,5] Both the lower segment of the cervical spine as well as the upper are strengthened and supported by a network of muscles, tendons, ligaments, and other structures.

Ligaments

Ligaments play a major role in the biomechanics of the cervical spine. The anterior longitudinal ligament limits hyperextension and forward movement.[8,9] It extends from the occipital bone and the anterior tubercle of the atlas all the way down to the sacrum, blending with the outer lamellae of the intervertebral disks and attaching to the ventral surface of the vertebrae as it passes between them. The posterior longitudinal ligament prevents hyperflexion.[8,9] It forms the anterior wall of the spinal canal and attaches to the dorsal surfaces of the vertebral bodies, extending from the occipital bone to the coccyx. The supraspinal ligament connects the apices of the spinous processes and resists spinal separation and flexion.[9] Intertransverse and capsular ligaments limit lateral bending[9] by connecting the transverse processes of adjacent vertebrae and padding the articulate capsules that surround and cushion the vertebral bones. The ligamentum flavum maintains constant disk tension, elongating with flexion and shortening with extension.[9] Although they are only thinly developed in the cervical spine, the membranous fibers of interspinal ligaments prevent excessive rotation,[9] as they connect adjoining spinous processes, extending from the root to the apex of each process.

Muscles

Muscles are dynamic stabilizers that function by moving the head and neck through controlled contractions. The splenius capitis and cervicis are deep muscles in the back used to extend the head and neck and to laterally flex and rotate the head to the same side with unilateral contraction.[9] The semispinalis capitis (complexus), semispinalis cervicis, and spinalis cervicis are muscles connected to thoracic vertebrae that extend and laterally flex and rotate the head and neck toward the side opposite the contraction.[9] Other muscles that move the head and neck include the trapezius, the sternocleidomastoid, and the anterior/middle scalenes.[9]

Other Stabilizers

In addition to the those mentioned previously, other support mechanisms include intervertebral disks, zygapophyseal joint capsules, and uncovertebral joints.[9] Between each pair of vertebrae (except for the atlas and the axis), there are small disks made of an inner gelatinous material called nucleus pulposus, encased by an outer ring called the annulus fibrosis.[5,8,9] These intervertebral disks act as fibrocartilaginous joints, enabling slight movement between vertebrae, but they also act as cushiony ligaments, holding the spine together comfortably. They play a crucial role as shock absorbers in the spine.[4] Zygapophyseal (facet) joint capsules are synovial joints located between the articular processes of each vertebrae.[5,9] In the cervical spine, they help to restrain forward translation. Finally, the uncovertebral joints are not true synovial joints, but arising from the posterolateral margins of the vertebral bodies in C3 to C7.[9]

Lordosis

When the cervical spine is properly aligned by all of these structures, it assumes a natural lordotic curve[8]; however, when the chin is lowered and the neck is flexed to 30° or more, the normal lordotic curve flattens out and the cervical spine converts into a segmented column.[5,8] In this position, the extra elasticity provided by the loose spacing of the vertebrae is lost.[1,4] Forces applied to the top of the head are now directed straight down the spinal column[8] instead of dissipating correctly through the network of paravertebral musculature, intervertebral disks, and the normal lordotic curve of the cervical spine.[5]

Injury Patterns

Although uncommon, both fatal and severe, nonfatal brain and spine injuries can occur during sports-related activities. These injuries have been noted in contact sports, such as football, ice hockey, wrestling, and rugby, as well as in noncontact sports like cheerleading, swimming and diving, baseball, equestrian, gymnastics, pole vault, rodeo, snowboarding, and skiing. Patterns exist in brain and cervical spine injuries that vary with each sport. Understanding these patterns is essential in prevention and recognition of injuries.[10]

Hyperflexion or hyperextension of the cervical spine in an athlete with a developmental or congenitally narrow spinal canal may cause neurologic injury by a pincer mechanism.[11] External forces that cause a combination of side bending and extension may lead to neuroforaminal compression or stretching, leading to injury of one or multiple cervical nerve roots. This is the mechanism involved with the injury known as a burner or stinger. Acceleration or deceleration forces that occur in whiplash injuries commonly cause injury to the muscle, ligamentous supports, or cervical facet joints.[12]

Among all sports, football has the highest number of catastrophic brain and cervical spine injuries.[13] A review of 1300 cervical spine injuries from the National Football Head and Neck Injury Registry has documented axial loading as the major mechanism of catastrophic cervical spine injuries.[14] In the normal cervical spine, the natural lordosis of the vertebral arch is able to tolerate substantial force by dissipating forces evenly across multiple levels. When the neck is flexed forward 30°, however, it becomes a straight segmented column that does not dissipate forces equally. Axial loading with the neck in a flexed position can then result in excessive forces on the vertebral bodies, leading to fractures and SCIs.[15] This is referred to as "spear tackling," and has been banned from football, although these injuries do continue to occur.

Although the number of catastrophic cervical spine injuries in ice hockey is low compared with other sports, the incidence per 1000 participants remains relatively high.[16] The typical mechanism of injury is axial loading caused by a blow to the head from collision with the boards, other players, the ice, or the goal post.[17] Most of these injuries occur when the injured player is checked from behind, causing the athlete to be thrown horizontally into the boards.[18]

Differential Diagnosis

See **Table 1**.

Examination

The physical examination of the neck with a suspected injury should focus on several elements. Visual inspection should be made of the spinal curvature, evaluating for ecchymosis or erythema, lacerations, and obvious deformities. The examiner should palpate for deformities, step-offs, and midline or paraspinal tenderness. Active and passive range of motion should be tested for flexion, extension, side bending, and rotation. Strength testing should be examined manually for bilateral upper and lower extremities. Sensation should be tested in all cervical dermatomes. Reflexes should be tested for at C5 (biceps), C6 (brachioradialis), C6/7 (pronator), and C7 (triceps),

Table 1 Differential diagnosis	
Cervical muscle strain	Injury to soft tissue of the neck, specifically a muscle or tendon.
Cervical ligament sprain	Injury to a ligamentous support of the cervical spine.
Cervical spine fracture	Injury to the bony structures of the cervical spine, specifically the vertebral body or vertebral processes.
Herniated disk	Herniation of the intervertebral disk, causing nerve root compression.
Transient quadriplegia	Neuropraxia causing bilateral burning or tingling pain, loss of strength, or loss of sensation, usually lasting <15 min but potentially as long as 48 h.
Cervical radiculopathy (burner/stinger)	Traction on the cervical nerve roots, causing unilateral shoulder/arm burning or stinging.
Cervical cord injury	Most catastrophic of spinal cord injuries, often leading to partial paralysis, complete paralysis, or death.
Nonorthopedic causes	Cardiovascular, endocrine, pulmonary, infectious.

L4 (patellar), L5 (medial hamstring), and S1 (Achilles), as well as pathologic reflexes with the Hoffman and Babinski reflex tests. Special tests such as the Spurling and Lhermitte should be performed as well.[12]

In the setting of acute trauma, a physician and/or certified athletic trainer with skills in the acute management of cervical spine injuries should evaluate and treat the patient. Focus should be placed on cervical stabilization. Although the lead rescuer is maintaining stability, another rescuer should make a primary assessment of airway, breathing, and circulation. If no further emergencies require immediate action, then secondary assessment may proceed. The second rescuer should palpate for normal curvature, deformities, lacerations, step-offs, and tenderness to bone or soft tissue. The second rescuer also should perform a neurologic examination of the athlete. This should be composed of motor and sensation testing, as well as a mental status assessment. If an athlete is unconscious or if assessment is limited, a cervical cord injury should be assumed.

Imaging
Many studies have helped determine whether or not to perform imaging. The National Emergency X-Radiography Utilization Study (NEXUS) criteria and Canadian Cervical Spine Rule (CCR) have been established to guide use of cervical spine radiography in patients with trauma. For alert patients with trauma, the CCR is superior to the NEXUS with respect of sensitivity and specificity for cervical spine injury (**Figs. 1** and **2**).[19,20]

If imaging is indicated, plain radiographs are an appropriate initial study to evaluate for bony anatomy and instability. Radiographs should include anteroposterior, lateral, and open-mouth (Odontoid) views. Flexion and extension views may be ordered to evaluate for abnormal segmental motion, ligamentous laxity, or atlantoaxial instability. The Torg-Pavlov ratio compares the diameter of the spinal canal to that of the vertebral body, and can be measured in the lateral view. A ratio of less than 0.8 is used to predict cervical stenosis, although its use is controversial and generally of historical significance only.

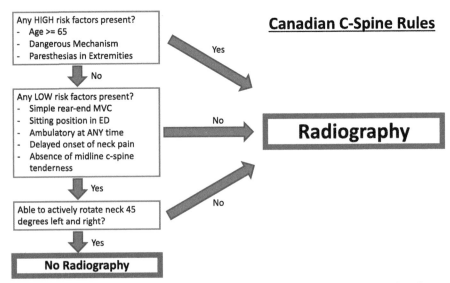

Fig. 1. Canadian cervical spine rule. ED, emergency department; MVC, motor vehicle collision.

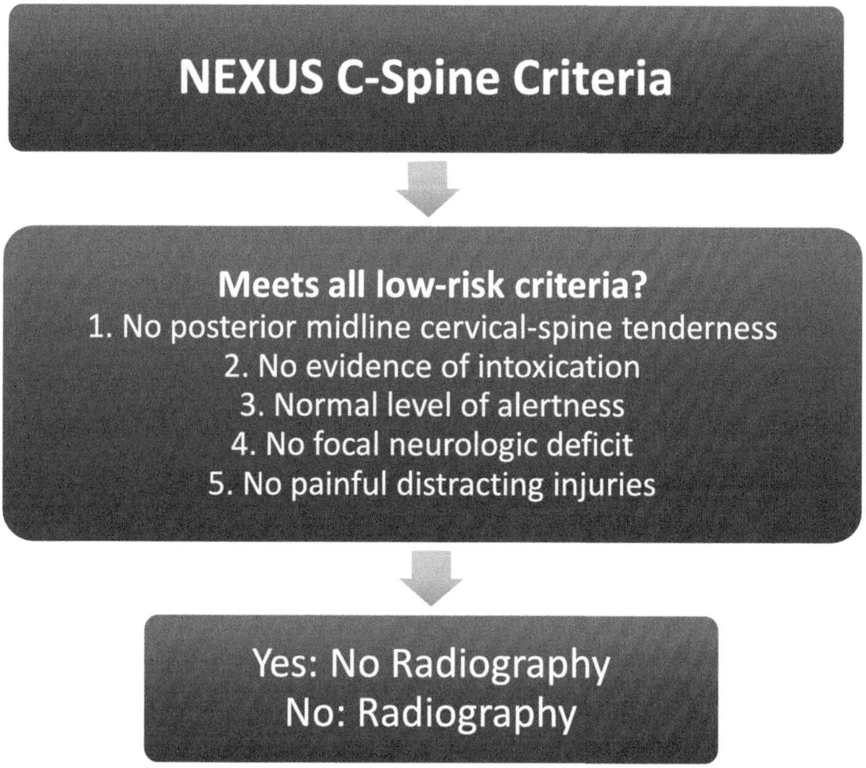

NEXUS C-Spine Criteria

Meets all low-risk criteria?
1. No posterior midline cervical-spine tenderness
2. No evidence of intoxication
3. Normal level of alertness
4. No focal neurologic deficit
5. No painful distracting injuries

Yes: No Radiography
No: Radiography

Fig. 2. National Emergency X-Radiography Utilization Study C-spine criteria.

Computed tomography (CT) imaging is useful to evaluate for clinically suspected fracture or bony pathology when radiographs are negative or equivocal. CT imaging is superior to radiographs in detecting both clinically significant and insignificant cervical spine injuries, and is recommended as the imaging modality of choice in children.[21] CT allows for better visualization of bony detail. For patients with neurologic symptoms who are unable to undergo MRI, CT myelogram is a useful tool to evaluate for spinal stenosis or neural compression.

MRI is a useful imaging tool to evaluate for soft tissue injury, ligamentous disruption, or disk herniation. MRI is also used to evaluate for SCIs, such as cord compression, cord disruption, cord contusions, or nerve root impingement. MRI is also useful for cervical canal measurements and functional reserve, the protective cushioning of cerebrospinal fluid around the spinal cord.[12] MRI has been found to identify additional injuries in 23.6% of patients with a normal CT, although the clinical significance of these abnormal findings is uncertain in the setting of patients without neurologic abnormalities.[22]

Other testing
In patients with persistent motor or sensory abnormalities after a cervical spine injury, an electromyogram and Nerve Conduction Study can be a useful diagnostic test. This is performed in the outpatient clinic setting. It can be used to differentiate whether a lesion is at the nerve root, brachial plexus, or peripheral nerve.

Acute management

Traditional management of suspected neck injuries has typically focused on immobilization, taking the approach of prioritizing precautions to prevent any potential cervical spine movement, to minimize the chance of neurologic injury. This protocol generally involves the routine use of manual in-line stabilization, a rigid cervical collar, and often a rigid backboard/spineboard as well, in all suspected head and neck injuries, regardless of patient condition. Although this approach initially appears to provide the safest framework, in practice research suggests it may be causing more harm than good, and a more flexible protocol may lead to better overall outcomes.[23–27]

In general, patients with suspected neck injuries can be thought of as falling into 1 of 4 categories: uninjured or minor injury, stable cervical spine fractures, unstable cervical spine fractures with completed neurologic deficits, and unstable cervical spine fractures without or with incomplete neurologic deficits. An overwhelming majority of patients (96%) fall into the first category, whereas stable fractures make up approximately 3% of the total. Fewer than 1%, then, have unstable fractures that may potentially benefit from immobilization.[28,29] Even among patients who have unstable fractures, neurologic deficits are rare, and most of those happen immediately at the time of injury.[28] Deficits that develop only later are extremely rare, with 1 review finding only 41 such case reports in the literature. Of those, 30 had no identifiable trigger, and only 1 developed deficits after the removal of a cervical collar. In multiple cases, neurologic deficits actually developed after the application of a cervical collar, which can be especially dangerous in patients with preexisting cervical spine abnormalities, such as ankylosing spondylitis.[30–33]

Most patients, then, cannot benefit from the routine application of a cervical collar, and only stand to suffer harm from its use. Research has indeed shown that cervical collars lead to a number of complications, including long-term pain after use, increased intracranial pressure and decreased venous return, increased aspiration risk, pressure ulcers, decreased respiratory ability (as demonstrated by a 15% decreased in forced expiratory volume in 1 second with use of both a collar and backboard), increased intubation time, delays in treatment, and increased cost in materials and extra downstream testing to "clear" the collar.[34–36]

Cervical spine immobilization is also likely the wrong goal as an approach as well. A correctly fitted cervical collar will allow 30° of flexion/extension, 16° of lateral bending, and 27° of rotation, and cadaveric studies have shown that they do not reduce c-spine movement in cadavers with unstable fractures.[37] Even internal fixation does not eliminate all movement, and the goal of acute management should aim at spinal motion restriction rather than full immobilization. Cervical spine injuries typically require more than 2000 to 6000 N of force, whereas a 4-kg head left hanging free to gravity will generate only 40 N. In addition, awake patients with injuries will typically protect their necks spontaneously, and it is unlikely that small, low-speed movements are enough to cause additional injury.[38,39] In fact, studies have shown that nonimmobilized patients do not have worse neurologic outcomes than those who were immobilized.[28]

A more commonsense, individualized approach has been proposed, aimed at limiting spinal motion and protecting the patient in transport without attempts at full immobilization. This approach calls for special attention and a more conservative management plan for patients with altered mental status or existing neurologic symptoms, but would allow for awake, alert patients with no neurologic deficits to be transported in a position of comfort (**Table 2**).[23–25,27]

Table 2 Spinal immobilization				
Patient Condition	No Neck Pain or Tenderness	Neck Pain or Tenderness	Neuro Signs or Symptoms	Altered Mental Status
Ambulatory	Position of comfort	Gurney position of comfort with/without support	Full	Position of comfort
Nonambulatory	Position of comfort	Gurney supine position of comfort with extrication support	Full	Full

Treatment

Treatment of acute neck injuries will vary based on the severity of the underlying injury. Soft tissue and peripheral nerve injuries such as stingers are generally self-limiting. For these injuries, rest, ice, nonsteroidal anti-inflammatories, and targeted physical therapy can help with recovery. A soft cervical collar has not been shown to provide any benefit, and may actually lead to stiffness and delayed recovery. Fractures should be referred to an orthopedic or neurosurgical spine specialist for definitive treatment.

Return to play

Return to play should focus on the safety of the athlete and his or her ability to avoid further injury. The severity of the injury will generally guide the timeline for full return. Soft tissue and muscle injuries are generally self-limiting, and most athletes will be allowed to return as tolerated. With minor neurologic injuries, such as stingers, athletes must be able to demonstrate full strength and range of motion of their neck and any other affected body part before being allowed to return to play. They must have a completely normal neurologic examination, and not have had bilateral symptoms, which would raise suspicion for a potential spinal cord injury.[40]

Some fractures, such as spinous process or unilateral laminar fractures, do not cause instability and may require no treatment or only brief immobilization, and the athlete can be safely returned to play after healing. Other fractures carry higher risks with return to sport, however, and decisions should be made in conjunction with a spine surgeon.[40]

Return to play after transient quadriparesis and is controversial, and should be carefully considered on a case-by-case basis. Athletes may be able to return after an initial brief episode, once they regain full strength and function, but multiple or prolonged (>24 hours) episodes should prompt consideration of disqualification. Any athlete with a permanent neurologic injury should be prohibited from further competition in regular contact sports; however, there are some lower intensity or noncontact sports, as well as sports designed for those with disabilities, in which they may participate safely.[40]

DISCLOSURE

The authors have nothing to disclose.

REFERENCES

1. Cooper MT, Mcgee KM, Anderson DG. Epidemiology of athletic head and neck injuries. In: Anderson DG, Helm GA, editors. Clinics in sports medicine. 2003.

p. 427–43. https://doi.org/10.1016/s0278-5919(02)00110-2, 22(3), head and neck injuries in sports medicine.

2. May JA, Crown LA, Geartner MC. Field-side emergencies. In: O'Connor FG, Casa DJ, Davis BA, et al, editors. ACSM's sports medicine: a comrehensive review. Philadelphia: Wolters Kluwer Health/Lippincott Williams & Wilkins; 2013. p. 84–91.

3. Bettencourt RB, Linder MM. Treatment of neck injuries. Prim Care 2013;40(2): 259–69.

4. Ghiselli G, Schaadt G, McAllister DR. On-the-field evaluation of an athlete with a head or neck injury. In: Anderson DG, Helm GA, editors. Clinics in sports medicine. 2003. p. 445–65. https://doi.org/10.1016/s0278-5919(02)00109-6, 22(3), Head and neck injuries in sports medicine.

5. Malagna GA, Hyman GS, Bowen JE, et al. Cervical spine. In: O'Connor FG, Casa DJ, Davis BA, et al, editors. ACSM's sports medicine: a comrehensive review. Philadelphia: Wolters Kluwer Health/Lippincott Williams & Wilkins; 2013. p. 292–6.

6. Yau RK, Kucera KL, Thomas LC, et al. Catastrophic sports injury research: thirty-fifth annual report, Fall 1984 - Spring 2017. 2018. Available at: https://nccsir.unc.edu/files/2018/09/NCCSIR-35th-Annual-All-Sport-Report-1982_2017_FINAL.pdf. Accessed March 22, 2019.

7. Snyder RL. Neck injuries. In: Madden CC, Putukian M, Young CC, et al, editors. Netter's sports medicine. Philadelphia: Saunders; 2010. p. 326–31.

8. McAlindon RJ. On field evaluation and management of head and neck injured athletes. In: Lauerman WC, editor. Clinics in sports medicine. 2002. p. 1–14. https://doi.org/10.1016/s0278-5919(03)00053-x, 21(1), the spine and sports.

9. Plastaras CT, Pang S. Cervical spine injuries and conditions. In: Harrast MA, Finnoff JT, editors. Sports medicine study guide and review for boards. New York: Demos Medical Publishing; 2012. p. 199–208.

10. Hutton MJ, McGuire RA, Dunn R, et al. Catastrophic cervical spine injuries in contact sports. Glob Spine J 2016;6:721–34.

11. McAlindon RJ. On field evaluation and management of head and neck injured athletes. Clin Sports Med 2002;21(1):1–14.

12. Malanga GA, Hyman GS, Bowen JE, et al. Cervical spine. ACSM's sports medicine a comprehensive review. Philadelphia: Wolters Kluwers Health/Lippincott Williams & Wilkin; 2013. p. 293–4 [Chapter 44].

13. Wolff C, Cantu R, Kucera K. Catastrophic neurologic injuries in sport. Handb Clin Neurol 2018;158:25–37 [Chapter 4].

14. Torg JS, Vegso JJ, O'Neil MJ, et al. The epidemiologic, pathologic, biomechanical, and cinematographic analysis of football-induced cervical spine trauma. Am J Sports Med 1990;18(1):50–7.

15. MacKnight JM, O'Connor FG, Casa DJ. Football. ACSM's sports medicine a comprehensive review. Philadelphia: Wolters Kluwers Health/Lippincott Williams & Wilkin; 2013. p. 630 [Chapter 92].

16. Mueller PO, Cantu RC. National center for catastrophic sports injury research: twentieth annual report. Fall 1982-spring 2002. Chapel Hill (NC): National Center for Catastrophic Sports Injury Research; 2002. p. 1–25.

17. Tator CH. Injuries in ice hockey: a recent, unsolved problem with many contributing factors. Clin Sports Med 1987;6(1):101–14.

18. Tator CH, Carson JD, Edmonds VE. Spinal injuries in ice hockey. Clin Sports Med 1998;17(1):183–94.

19. Stiell IG, Clement CM, McKnight RD, et al. The Canadian C-spine rule versus the NEXUS low-risk criteria in patients with trauma. N Engl J Med 2003;349(26): 2510–8.

20. Gopinathan NR, Viswanathan VK, Crawford AH. Cervical spine evaluation in pediatric trauma: a review and an update of current concepts. Indian J Orthop 2018; 52(5):489–500.

21. Hale AT, Alvarado A, Key AK, et al. X-ray vs. CT in identifying significant C-spine injuries in the pediatric population. Childs Nerv Syst 2017;33(11):1977–83.

22. Maung AA, Johnson DC, Barre K, et al. Cervical spine MRI in patients with negative CT: a prospective, multicenter study of the Research Consortium of New England Centers for Trauma (ReCONECT). J Trauma Acute Care Surg 2017;82(2): 263–9.

23. Stroh G, Braude D. Can an out-of-hospital cervical spine clearance protocol identify all patients with injuries? An argument for selective immobilization. Ann Emerg Med 2001;37(6):609–15.

24. Domeier R, Frederiksen S, Welch K. Prospective performance assessment of an out-of-hospital protocol for selective spine immobilization using clinical spine clearance criteria. Ann Emerg Med 2005;46(2):123–31.

25. Burton J, Dunn M, Harmon NR, et al. A statewide, prehospital emergency medical service selective patient spine immobilization protocol. J Trauma Acute Care Surg 2006;61(1):161–7.

26. Vaillancourt C, Charette M, Kasaboski A, et al. Evaluation of the safety of C-spine clearance by paramedics: design and methodology. BMC Emerg Med 2011; 11:1.

27. Sundstrøm T, Asbjørnsen H, Habiba S, et al. Prehospital use of cervical collars in trauma patients: a critical review. J Neurotrauma 2014;31(6):531–40.

28. Hauswald M, Ong G, Tandberg D, et al. Out-of-hospital spinal immobilization: its effect on neurologic injury. Acad Emerg Med 1998;5:214–9.

29. Rhee P, Kuncir EJ, Johnson L, et al. Cervical spine injury is highly dependent on the mechanism of injury following blunt and penetrating assault. J Trauma 2006; 61(1):166–70.

30. Ben-Galim P, Dreiangel N, Mattox KL, et al. Extrication collars can result in abnormal separation between vertebrae in the presence of a dissociative injury. J Trauma 2010;69(2):447–50.

31. Podolsky SM, Hoffman JR, Pietrafesa CA. Neurologic complications following immobilization of cervical spine fracture in a patient with ankylosing spondylitis. Ann Emerg Med 1983;12:578–80.

32. Papadopoulos MC, Chakraborty A, Waldron G, et al. Lesson of the week: exacerbating cervical spine injury by applying a hard collar. BMJ 1999;319:171–2.

33. Slagel SA, Skiendzielewski JJ, McMurry FG. Osteomyelitis of the cervical spine: reversible quadraplegia resulting from Philadelphia collar placement. Ann Emerg Med 1985;14:912–5.

34. Raphael JH, Chotai R. Effects of the cervical collar on cerebrospinal fluid pressure. Anaesthesia 1994;49:437–9.

35. Dodd FM, Simon E, McKeown D, et al. The effect of a cervical collar on the tidal volume of anaesthetised adult patients. Anaesthesia 1995;50:961–3.

36. Houghton DJ, Curley JW. Dysphagia caused by a hard cervical collar. Br J Neurosurg 1996;10:501–2.

37. Horodyski M, DiPaola CP, Conrad BP, et al. Cervical collars are insufficient for immobilizing an unstable cervical spine injury. J Emerg Med 2011;41(5):513–9.

38. Shafer J, Naunheim R, West J. Cervical spine motion during extrication: a pilot study. J Emerg Med 2009;10(2):74–8.
39. Conrad B, Marchese D, Rechtine GR, et al. Motion in the unstable cervical spine when transferring a patient positioned prone to a spine board. J Athl Train 2013; 48(6):797–803.
40. Cantu RC, Li YM, Abdulhamid M, et al. Return to play after cervical spine injury in sports. Curr Sports Med Rep 2013;12(1):14–7.

Acute Sports-Related Head Injuries

Stephen M. Carek, MD, CAQSM[a],*, James R. Clugston, MD, MS, CAQSM[b]

KEYWORDS

- Head trauma • Sports-related concussion • Persistent postconcussive symptoms
- Epidural hematoma • Subdural hemorrhage • Intracerebral hemorrhage
- Diffuse axonal injury

KEY POINTS

- Although sports-related concussion is common, there are several other types of head injuries that can present similarly but rapidly worsen necessitating rapid identification and escalation of care.
- Although rare, epidural hematomas, subdural hemorrhages, intracerebral hemorrhage, diffuse axonal injury, and second impact syndrome are all significant pathologies that should be excluded when evaluating a patient with suspected head injury.
- A high suspicion for, and a low threshold for, removing an athlete from play after a suspected head injury should be maintained in sideline settings.
- Diagnosis of concussion on the sideline remains challenging. Evaluations should be multimodal in nature and include continued observation, as symptoms can develop or worsen over time.
- Management of concussion has evolved over the past several years, with a more active, but symptom-limited, approach now viewed as beneficial for most patients in expediting recovery and decreasing overall symptom burden.

INTRODUCTION

Head injuries are commonly encountered in sport and are routinely evaluated by primary care physicians. They can have a wide range of presentations, from nonspecific signs to obvious symptoms and can include focal neurologic deficits, cervical spine injury, and acute vascular conditions. Sports-related head injuries accounted for 1.7 million emergency department (ED) visits from 2007 to 2011, with 38% occurring in

[a] Department of Family Medicine, University of South Carolina, School of Medicine–Greenville, Center for Family Medicine - Greenville, 877 West Faris Road, Greenville, SC 29605, USA;
[b] Department of Community Health & Family Medicine and Department of Neurology, University Athletic Association University of Florida, UF Student Health Care Center, 280 Fletcher Dr | PO Box 117500, Gainesville, FL 32611-7500, USA
* Corresponding author.
E-mail address: Stephen.carek@prismahealth.org

Prim Care Clin Office Pract 47 (2020) 177–188
https://doi.org/10.1016/j.pop.2019.10.010
0095-4543/20/© 2019 Elsevier Inc. All rights reserved.
primarycare.theclinics.com

children 12 to 17 years of age and 79% in patients younger than or equal to 24 years. In collegiate sports, head and neck injuries account for 12.8% of practice-related injuries and 9.8% of game injuries across all genders and sports.[1] Rugby, ice hockey, and American football have the most ED visits for head trauma of all organized sports.[2] Head injuries may also go unreported due to an athlete's misconception that the injury is not severe enough to mention it to medical staff or due to deliberate hiding of the condition to avoid disqualification. Head injuries are typically the result of either direct or indirect contact with forces transmitted to the brain and the consequence of these neurologic injuries has a potentially high incidence of morbidity and mortality depending on the forces experienced (location and magnitude) and individual susceptibility. It is estimated that up to 70% of traumatic deaths and 20% of permanent disability in sports are due to head and neck injuries, with football being the most common sport with head trauma–related deaths.[3,4]

It is important that physicians involved in sports-related care understand the spectrum of head injuries and their management. This article begins by describing potential catastrophic head injuries from sport, as although they are rare, it is imperative for physicians to recognize these urgent conditions and institute appropriate initial management to increase survival and decrease morbidity. The focus then turns to the most common head injury in sport, sports-related concussion (SRC), which although considered a "mild" type of traumatic brain injury, may produce significant morbidity and has garnered significant public attention and research interest in recent years.

POTENTIAL CATASTROPHIC HEAD INJURIES
Epidural Hematoma

Epidural hematoma is the accumulation of blood between the dura and the skull. Typically caused by an acceleration-deceleration head injury, the mechanism of injury can result in inward deformity leading to dural detachment from the inner table of the skull. Most patients with an epidural hematoma have a skull fracture, which damages the middle meningeal artery or vein. In addition, bleeding can occur from the actual bone fragments, leading to a collection of blood within the epidural space, which results in a classic biconvex shape of hematoma seen on computed tomography (CT).

An important distinguishing feature of this clinical entity is the "lucid interval." The lucid interval occurs when a substantial blow sustained to the cranium can potentially cause the patient to briefly lose consciousness or be temporarily altered, but the patient may subsequently seem asymptomatic for several minutes to hours. The trauma to the skull or dural vessels leads to a slow accumulation of blood in the epidural space. This hematoma may ultimately reach a critically large size, increasing the intracranial pressure and resulting in lateralized shift of the brain, uncal herniation, anisocoria, decreased consciousness, and potentially death. The condition is typically diagnosed when worsening symptoms or focal neurologic deficits are seen and head CT is performed. Patients with an epidural hematoma and neurologic symptoms require an emergency craniotomy for evacuation of the hematoma to reduce intracranial pressure. Early identification and surgical decompression correlates with improved survival, whereas high hematoma volume and midline displacement correlates with poorer outcomes.[5] It is imperative that frequent serial monitoring during the ensuing hours after an injury be performed to identify this deterioration suggestive of this and other severe brain injuries.

Subdural Hemorrhage

Subdural hemorrhages are more frequent than epidural hematomas and are the leading cause of catastrophic death in high school and collegiate football players,[6] occurring at a rate of around 6.5 per year in US high school football.[3] These occur when the bridging veins between the brain and the dura are torn, leading to the pooling of blood into a potential space. They are classified as acute (within 24 hours), subacute (24 hours–2 weeks), and chronic (over 2 weeks). The athlete with an acute subdural hematoma is usually unconscious, but presentation can vary and includes those who are awake and alert with no focal neurologic deficits, but who subsequently experience declining mental status, headache, anisocoria, or loss of consciousness. In a subdural hemorrhage, the magnitude of impact directly correlates to the degree of parenchymal damage and if great enough may result in a fatal injury.

CT scanning can identify a subdural hemorrhage in the acute setting, with a crescent-shaped, hyperdense mass appearing along the convexity of the skull. Several case studies have implicated recent concussion or head injury before the inciting impact leading to a subdural hemorrhage.[7-10] With acute subdural hemorrhages, rapid progression and deterioration of mental status requires immediate neurosurgical evaluation and consideration for surgical evacuation. Occasionally, subdural hematomas may develop slowly over a period of days to weeks, in which case symptoms are often vague and may resemble those of a mild traumatic brain injury; however, they may also have subtle mental, motor, or sensory signs and symptoms.

Intracerebral Hemorrhage

An intracerebral hemorrhage is another form of intracranial hemorrhage seen after head trauma. This injury represents direct bleeding in the brain parenchyma, typically from a torn artery or small caliber arteriole. The mechanism is typically a tensile or shearing force that stretches the brain, as in a coup or countercoup injury. Intracerebral hemorrhages are not typically associated with a lucid interval and presentations can vary greatly, depending on the location and extent of hemorrhagic lesions. Initial symptoms include headache, confusion, retrograde amnesia, and focal deficits correlating to the area of injury but may progress to further neurologic deterioration, including coma and death.[11] Following the acute event, worsening mass effect can occur due to delayed intracerebral hemorrhage or edema, requiring continued clinical monitoring with serial examinations. CT of the brain demonstrates a hyperdense lesion within the brain parenchyma, typically occurring at the frontal or temporal poles. Surgical intervention for decompression is warranted in patients with signs of increasing intracranial pressure or a decline in neurologic status, whereas small intracerebral hemorrhages can be managed nonoperatively if the patient remains neurologically stable.

Diffuse Axonal Injury

Diffuse axonal injury (DAI) is a diffuse axonal disruption of white matter in the cortex and brainstem. Excessive strain of white matter and associated small blood vessels is created from sudden rotational acceleration, which can potentially cause axotomy or hemorrhage. DAI commonly occurs at the gray-white matter junction and where long white matter tracts are located, such as the corpus callosum, internal capsule, cerebral white matter, fornix, midbrain, pons, medulla, and cerebellum. Instant axonal tearing can initiate a cascade of events, which cause changes in lipid membrane permeability, ion shifts, excessive neurotransmitter release, hypoxia, free radical formation, and activation of inflammatory cells. Disruption of axonal neurofilament organization occurs and impairs axonal transport leading to axonal swelling, Wallerian degeneration, and transection.[12] Because of the microscopic nature of this injury pattern, initial CT or MRI of the brain may be unremarkable. In this case, diffusion weighted imaging is more sensitive for DAI than conventional CT and MRI.[13]

A patient who has sustained a DAI typically presents in a coma and may exhibit decorticate or decerebrate posturing, severe posttraumatic amnesia, and cognitive deficits after awakening. Treatment is supportive during coma with medical or surgical treatment as needed for signs and symptoms of increased intracranial pressures. These types of injuries are relatively rare in organized, nonvehicular sports and outcomes are difficult to predict but range from extensive chronic disability to complete clinical recovery.[14]

Second Impact Syndrome

Second impact syndrome occurs when a second concussive event occurs before recovery from an initial concussion, with subsequent change in mental status and possible catastrophic neurologic injury.[15] There has been some debate regarding the existence and precise definition of second impact syndrome,[16,17] most stemming from the rarity of this type of event. Controversy exists regarding whether the cerebral edema that develops is truly due to a second hit or is a progression from the previous hit; how far apart the first and second hits can be; whether subdural hematomas or other structural injuries play a significant role in the progression to severe edema; and why there is a paucity of cases reported outside the United States.[15] There is some thought that the pathophysiology of second impact syndrome involves a loss of autoregulation of the brain's blood supply, leading to vascular engorgement, marked increase in intracranial pressure, brain herniation, and ultimately coma or death. Current identified risk factors for second impact syndrome include participation in boxing and American football, male gender, and young age, with most of the cases reported in the teenage years[15]

SPORTS-RELATED CONCUSSION

Concussions or mild traumatic brain injuries are the most common type of head injury encountered in sports settings and have become a widely researched and publicly discussed topic. Referred to as SRCs, they occur during sport as a result of traumatic biomechanical forces to the brain, either by a direct blow to the head, face, or neck or by an indirect impact elsewhere on the body that transmits to the brain. These typically result in the rapid onset of short-lived impairment of neurologic function that typically resolves over days to weeks. The Center for Disease Control and Prevention estimates that there are between 1.6 and 3.8 million recreation-related concussive injuries annually in the United States and rates of reported concussions have increased significantly over the past decade.[18–20] Concussions, both sport and nonsport related, may occur across the typical human life span, but the majority occurs during childhood and adolescence.[21] There continues to be large barriers to identifying and understanding the importance of concussions, as up to 50% of concussions sustained by children may not be reported to any health care provider.[22] High-risk contact sports, including American-style football, hockey, and soccer are associated with increased rates of SRC. In sports with similar rules for men and women, such as basketball and soccer, female athletes have higher rates of SRC and time loss for recovery as compared with their male counterparts.[23,24]

On-Field Management and Sideline Assessment

Recognition and evaluation of SRC is challenging due to its sometimes subtle presentation and its potentially evolving nature. Initial on-field or sideline evaluation of an athlete suspected of sustaining a traumatic head injury must include assessment of the airway, breathing, and cardiac function. If a cervical spine injury is suspected, spinal precautions must be initiated. Emergency transfer should occur if there are signs of a more serious brain injury, such as deteriorating mental status, focal neurologic findings (abnormal or unequal pupil reaction, abnormalities with extraocular movements, gross abnormalities on screening motor/sensory examination), or acutely worsening symptoms. Once potential catastrophic injuries have been excluded, the athlete should continue to be held from play and undergo further evaluation. Protecting the athlete from additional head trauma and exertion is vital if concussion is suspected due to potential for acute and long-term sequelae. Immediate identification and removal from competition is important, as delayed identification is associated with a prolonged duration of symptoms and more time missed from sport.[25] The athlete should be assessed by a licensed health care provider trained in the evaluation and management of concussion.[26] Most of the SRCs occur without a loss of consciousness or frank neurologic signs, and there is no perfect diagnostic test or marker that can reliably diagnose all SRCs in the acute setting. Instead the assessment is clinically based, relying heavily on symptom report and physical examination, and often includes functional concussion assessment tools as mentioned later. As SRC symptoms may be delayed and/or evolve, serial evaluations during the acute stages are necessary.

Concussion Assessment Tools

Multifunctional sideline evaluations are helpful in determining if an athlete has sustained a concussion. Several brief symptom assessments as well as cognitive, balance, and vision tests have been developed to rapidly assess functions that are frequently diminished after concussion. These tests are typically administered by a provider with experience in concussion management, such as a certified athletic trainer or team physician. The Sport Concussion Assessment Tool (SCAT), first developed in 2004 by the Concussion in Sports Group combined several approaches to concussion assessment, including symptoms, cognitive status, balance, and gross neurologic functioning.[27] This has undergone several revisions, with the most recent iteration, the SCAT5, introduced in 2016 as a tool for the evaluation of individuals 13 years or older suspected of having sustained an SRC.[28] For children aged 5 to 12 years, the Child SCAT5 was developed, which includes more child-friendly language and areas for parents to report observed symptoms.[29] The SCAT5 includes immediate acute assessment with background and demographic information. There are 8 components of the SCAT5, including Glasgow Coma Scale, Maddocks questions, symptoms checklist, modified Standardized Assessment of Concussion (SAC), neck examination, and modified Balance Error Scoring System (BESS).[30] The Maddocks questions consist of 5 simple questions about the current athletic event, which aim to evaluate short- and intermediate-term memory. The symptoms checklist consists of 22 common concussion-related symptoms that are scaled from 0 (none) to 6 (severe).[30] The modified SAC test evaluates 4 neurocognitive domains: orientation, memory, concentration, and delayed recall. The physical examination evaluates the neck for range of motion, tenderness, extremity strength, and sensation. Postural stability or balance is assessed using either the modified BESS or the tandem gait test.

In recent years, tests involving the visio-vestibular and ocular motor systems have been advocated for inclusion during the initial evaluation of concussion. Maneuvers from the vestibular ocular motor screen originally developed for in-office follow-up are being incorporated in the sideline physical examination. The King-Devick (KD) test, a proprietary test of rapid number naming involving saccadic eye movements, has also been increasingly used in acute settings.[31,32] It can be administered in less than 2 minutes and consists of 3 successive test cards, with single digit numbers, variably spaced both horizontally and vertically. The KD test requires prior testing (baseline) before suspected injury to provide a comparison for postinjury results.[33] An appreciation for learning effects and the influence of motivation differences between postinjury and baseline settings is helpful when interpreting these tests.

Sideline Management and Disposition

When a player is being evaluated for, or has been diagnosed with, an SRC, a good safety strategy is to confiscate an integral piece of equipment to prevent an inadvertent return to the game or practice.[26] A concussed player should be removed from play and serially monitored for deteriorating physical or mental status. If after a full sideline assessment the diagnosis of concussion is not thought to have occurred and the player is allowed to continue playing, serial evaluations should still be performed to ensure the correct decision was made.[26] If an athlete is diagnosed with SRC, they should be monitored for a period of time and if there are no signs of deterioration, may be allowed to return home provided they have received instructions for typical follow-up with a provider experienced in management of SRC and also education on when to seek emergency care and what signs and symptoms might trigger the need for such care. Providing this information in both an oral and a written format to the athlete as well as friends and family is preferred.

There is a paucity of evidence that any particular medication is effective in treating the acute symptoms of concussion and treatment should be based on common approaches to each specific symptom. Consideration for medications that affect the central nervous system, such as antidepressants, stimulants, and certain antinausea medications, should be made, as they may cloud the follow-up symptom report and cognitive examination. Treatment of headache initially after concussion is limited to acetaminophen, as it offers possible benefit without significant increased bleeding risk or rebound headache compared with nonsteroidal antiinflammatory drugs (NSAIDs). Typically, if after 24 to 48 hours there has been no development of neurologic symptoms, NSAIDs for headache may be started. A brief period of cognitive and physical rest immediately after the injury is recommended as symptoms abate, but as will be mentioned in a later section, light, nonsymptom provoking aerobic activity may be safely attempted after this period and is now thought to benefit recovery in many instances. However, it is important to refrain from intensive training and contact or collision activities, which may significantly worsen symptoms in the early postinjury phase.

Follow-up Management

There is accumulating evidence that extended rest postinjury does not improve outcome and may increase symptoms.[34] Recent evidence suggests that early initiation (within a week of injury) of active rehabilitation, including light aerobic exercise, is associated with shorter returns to sport, school, and work.[35,36] An active treatment plan that focuses on physical therapy, vestibular therapy, and or subsymptom threshold exercise may improve recovery from concussion if they are implemented at the right time.[37] Most adult athletes and pediatric athletes will have complete recovery from symptoms within 1 to 2 weeks and 3 to 4 weeks, respectively.[38] However, some do not and several factors may contribute to prolonged recovery including early posttraumatic headache, symptoms of fatigue/fogginess, early amnesia, younger age/level of play, and persistent neurocognitive impairments on follow-up testing.[39]

Symptoms that persist for greater than 2 weeks in adults and greater than 4 weeks in children are referred to persistent postconcussive symptoms.[36] Several domains of symptoms can be managed with medical and nonmedication-based therapies, which are described further in **Fig. 1**. Although there are no current medications indicated for treating concussion, treatments can focus on symptom management with the same medications used in patients without a concussion.[40] Ongoing follow-up should be tailored to individual patients with determination of return to play, return to drive, and return to work guided by symptomatic and functional improvement. Successfully returning to academic settings typically is helped by a gradual resumption of activity and may require academic

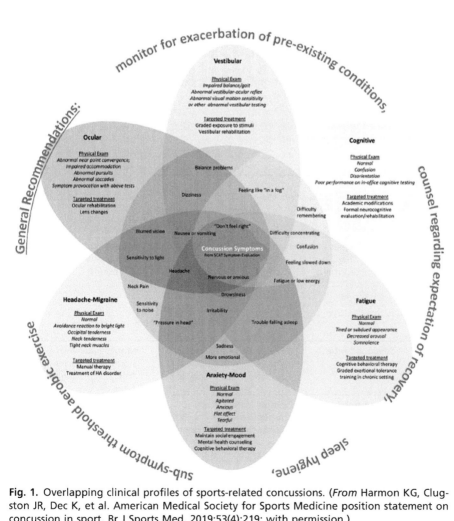

Fig. 1. Overlapping clinical profiles of sports-related concussions. (*From* Harmon KG, Clugston JR, Dec K, et al. American Medical Society for Sports Medicine position statement on concussion in sport. Br J Sports Med. 2019;53(4):219; with permission.)

Table 1
Graduated return to sport protocol

Stage	Activity	Goal	Requirement for Progression
1	Physical and cognitive rest	Recovery	Asymptomatic for 24 h
2	Light aerobic activity	Increase heart rate	Heart rate <70% of maximum while remaining asymptomatic
3	Sports-specific exercise	Increase body movement	Remain asymptomatic
4	Noncontact training drills	Exercise, coordination, and cognitive load	Remain asymptomatic and increase functions
5	Full-contact practice	Restore athlete's confidence and assess functional skills	If asymptomatic, may obtain medical clearance for return to competition
6	Return to play	—	—

Data from Refs.[27,37,50,51]

modifications, including a reduced workload, shortened school or work days, and frequent breaks to allow provoked symptoms to improve.[41] Several protocols exist to guide a gradual return to sport and learn/work programs as the patient's symptoms resolve. These stepwise programs (**Tables 1** and **2**), should be monitored with a professional experienced in concussion management. If any symptoms develop during the protocol, the patient typically returns to the previous asymptomatic step and may attempt progression after 24 hours.

Table 2
Graduated return to school/work protocol

Stage	Activity	Goal	Requirement for Progression
1	Daily activities at home that do not exacerbate the child's symptoms	Typical activities of the child during the day as long as they do not increase symptoms (eg, reading, texting, screen time). Start with 5–15 min at a time and gradually build up	Gradual return to typical activities without symptoms
2	School activities	Homework, reading, or other cognitive activities outside of the classroom	Asymptomatic with homework, increase tolerance to cognitive work
3	Return to school part-time	Gradual introduction of schoolwork. May need to start with a partial school day or with increased breaks during the day	Asymptomatic with partial school day, increased school activities
4	Return to school full-time	Gradually progress school activities until a full day can be tolerated	Return to full academic activities and catch up on missed work

Data from Refs.[41,49,50]

Postconcussion Syndrome

In some cases, concussion symptoms can be prolonged. This persistence of symptoms for more than 3 months from injury is referred to as "postconcussion syndrome." This diagnosis included a history of head trauma with a constellation of nonspecific symptoms, including headache, dizziness, malaise, fatigue, mood changes, decreased concentration, and insomnia.[42] There is controversy existing regarding this clinical entity and no well-defined treatment strategies exist,[26] although active rehabilitation strategies and cognitive behavioral therapy may be effective in the treatment of postconcussion syndrome.[37,43,44] Factors that may contribute to prolonged recovery from concussion include preexisting psychiatric conditions or athletes who continue in competition after sustaining a concussion.[25,45,46] Similar to the management of concussion, patients with postconcussion syndrome require academic and workplace accommodations that are adapted as symptoms resolve. Serial tracking of symptoms and functional status is essential after an injury because psychosocial factors may confound symptoms and recovery over time. Vestibular therapy has proved to be beneficial for athletes suffering from persistent dizziness or cervicogenic dysfunction following a concussion.[47] Cognitive behavioral therapy may help with emotional struggles or sleep-related issues related to a concussion.[43,48]

SUMMARY

Head injuries from sport participation, while commonly encountered by primary care providers, are often challenging to diagnose. An appropriate clinical evaluation, shortly after a reported head injury, is critical to identify clinical deterioration or initiate escalation of care. Although rare, epidural hematomas, subdural hemorrhages, intracerebral hemorrhage, DAI, and second impact syndrome are all significant pathologies that should be excluded when evaluating a patient with suspected head injury. A provider should have a high suspicion for diagnosing and a low threshold for removing an athlete from play after a suspected head injury. Such athletes should be monitored closely and repeatedly. A typical evaluation for SRC is multimodal, including symptom report, neurologic examination, and additional testing of cognitive, balance, and vision function. Management of SRC continues to espouse avoidance of potential contact activities until successful completion of return to sport, learn, and work have been achieved, but early introduction of symptom-limited aerobic activity has gained favor.

DISCLOSURE

The authors have nothing to disclose.

REFERENCES

1. Hootman JM, Dick R, Agel J. Epidemiology of collegiate injuries for 15 sports: summary and recommendations for injury prevention initiatives. J Athl Train 2007;42(2):311–9.
2. Pfister T, Pfister K, Hagel B, et al. The incidence of concussion in youth sports: a systematic review and meta-analysis. Br J Sports Med 2016;50(5):292–7.
3. Boden BP, Tacchetti RL, Cantu RC, et al. Catastrophic head injuries in high school and college football players. Am J Sports Med 2007;35(7):1075–81.
4. Mueller F, Kucera K, Cox L. Catastrophic sports injury research: thirtieth annual report 1982-2012. Chapel Hill, NC: University of North Carolina; 2012. p. 1–64.
5. Rivas JJ, Lobato RD, Sarabia R, et al. Extradural hematoma: analysis of factors influencing the courses of 161 patients. Neurosurgery 1988;23(1):44–51.

6. Kucera KL, Yau RK, Register-Mihalik J, et al. Traumatic brain and spinal cord fatalities among high school and college football players - United States, 2005-2014. MMWR Morb Mortal Wkly Rep 2017;65(52):1465–9.

7. Kersey RD. Acute subdural hematoma after a reported mild concussion: a case report. J Athl Train 1998;33(3):264–8.

8. Yengo-Kahn AM, Gardner RM, Kuhn AW, et al. Sport-related structural brain injury: 3 cases of subdural hemorrhage in american high school football. World Neurosurg 2017;106:1055.e5-11.

9. Logan SM, Bell GW, Leonard JC. Acute subdural hematoma in a high school football player after 2 unreported episodes of head trauma: a case report. J Athl Train 2001;36(4):433–6.

10. Potts MA, Stewart EW, Griesser MJ, et al. Exceptional neurologic recovery in a teenage football player after second impact syndrome with a thin subdural hematoma. PM R 2012;4(7):530–2.

11. Bailes JE, Hudson V. Classification of sport-related head trauma: a spectrum of mild to severe injury. J Athl Train 2001;36(3):236–43.

12. Mckee AC, Daneshvar DH. The neuropathology of traumatic brain injury. Handb Clin Neurol 2015;127:45–66.

13. Huisman TA, Sorensen AG, Hergan K, et al. Diffusion-weighted imaging for the evaluation of diffuse axonal injury in closed head injury. J Comput Assist Tomogr 2003;27(1):5–11.

14. Humble SS, Wilson LD, Wang L, et al. Prognosis of diffuse axonal injury with traumatic brain injury. J Trauma Acute Care Surg 2018;85(1):155–9.

15. McLendon LA, Kralik SF, Grayson PA, et al. The controversial second impact syndrome: a review of the literature. Pediatr Neurol 2016;62:9–17.

16. Stovitz SD, Weseman JD, Hooks MC, et al. What definition is used to describe second impact syndrome in sports? a systematic and critical review. Curr Sports Med Rep 2017;16(1):50–5.

17. McCrory P. Does second impact syndrome exist? Clin J Sport Med 2001;11(3):144–9.

18. Rosenthal JA, Foraker RE, Collins CL, et al. National high school athlete concussion rates from 2005-2006 to 2011-2012. Am J Sports Med 2014;42(7):1710–5.

19. Centers for Disease Control and Prevention. Nonfatal traumatic brain injuries related to sports and recreation activities among persons aged ≤19 years–United States, 2001-2009. MMWR Morb Mortal Wkly Rep 2011;60(39):1337–42.

20. Zuckerman SL, Kerr ZY, Yengo-Kahn A, et al. Epidemiology of sports-related concussion in NCAA athletes from 2009-2010 to 2013-2014: incidence, recurrence, and mechanisms. Am J Sports Med 2015;43(11):2654–62.

21. Selassie AW, Wilson DA, Pickelsimer EE, et al. Incidence of sport-related traumatic brain injury and risk factors of severity: a population-based epidemiologic study. Ann Epidemiol 2013;23(12):750–6.

22. Bryan MA, Rowhani-Rahbar A, Comstock RD, et al. Sports- and recreation-related concussions in US youth. Pediatrics 2016;138(1) [pii:e20154635].

23. Covassin T, Swanik CB, Sachs ML. Sex differences and the incidence of concussions among collegiate athletes. J Athl Train 2003;38(3):238–44.

24. Covassin T, Moran R, Elbin RJ. Sex differences in reported concussion injury rates and time loss from participation: an update of the National Collegiate Athletic Association Injury Surveillance Program From 2004-2005 Through 2008-2009. J Athl Train 2016;51(3):189–94.

25. Asken BM, Bauer RM, Guskiewicz KM, et al. Immediate removal from activity after sport-related concussion is associated with shorter clinical recovery and less

severe symptoms in collegiate student-athletes. Am J Sports Med 2018;46(6): 1465–74.

26. Harmon KG, Drezner JA, Gammons M, et al. American Medical Society for Sports Medicine position statement: concussion in sport. Br J Sports Med 2013;47(1): 15–26.

27. McCrory P, Johnston K, Meeuwisse W, et al. Summary and agreement statement of the 2nd International Conference on Concussion in Sport, Prague 2004. Br J Sports Med 2005;39(4):196–204.

28. Echemendia RJ, Meeuwisse W, McCrory P, et al. The Sport Concussion Assessment Tool 5th Edition (SCAT5): Background and rationale. Br J Sports Med 2017; 51(11):848–50.

29. Davis GA, Purcell L, Schneider KJ, et al. The child sport concussion assessment tool 5th edition (child SCAT5): background and rationale. Br J Sports Med 2017; 51(11):859–61.

30. Davis GA, Echemendia RJ, Meeuwisse W, et al. The Sport Concussion Assessment Tool 5th Edition (SCAT5): Background and rationale. Br J Sports Med 2017;0:1–8. https://doi.org/10.1136/bjsports-2017-097506SCAT5.

31. Galetta KM, Liu M, Leong DF, et al. The King-Devick test of rapid number naming for concussion detection: meta-analysis and systematic review of the literature. Concussion 2016;1(2):CNC8.

32. Marinides Z, Galetta KM, Andrews CN, et al. Vision testing is additive to the sideline assessment of sports-related concussion. Neurol Clin Pract 2015;5(1):25–34.

33. Galetta KM, Brandes LE, Maki K, et al. The King-Devick test and sports-related concussion: study of a rapid visual screening tool in a collegiate cohort. J Neurol Sci 2011;309(1–2):34–9.

34. Thomas DG, Apps JN, Hoffmann RG, et al. Benefits of strict rest after acute concussion: a randomized controlled trial. Pediatrics 2015;135(2):213–23.

35. Lawrence DW, Richards D, Comper P, et al. Earlier time to aerobic exercise is associated with faster recovery following acute sport concussion. PLoS One 2018;13(4):e0196062.

36. Harmon KG, Clugston JR, Dec K, et al. American Medical Society for Sports Medicine position statement on concussion in sport. Br J Sports Med 2019;53(4): 213–25.

37. Leddy JJ, Baker JG, Willer B. Active rehabilitation of concussion and postconcussion syndrome. Phys Med Rehabil Clin N Am 2016;27(2):437–54.

38. Henry LC, Elbin RJ, Collins MW, et al. Examining recovery trajectories after sport-related concussion with a multimodal clinical assessment approach. Neurosurgery 2016;78(2):232–41.

39. Giza CC, Kutcher JS, Ashwal S, et al. Summary of evidence-based guideline update: evaluation and management of concussion in sports: report of the Guideline Development Subcommittee of the American Academy of Neurology. Neurology 2013;80(24):2250–7.

40. Scorza KA, Cole W. Current concepts in concussion: initial evaluation and management. Am Fam Physician 2019;99(7):426–34.

41. Master CL, Mayer AR, Quinn D, et al. Concussion. Ann Intern Med 2018;169(1): ITC1–16.

42. Quinn DK, Mayer AR, Master CL, et al. Prolonged postconcussive symptoms. Am J Psychiatry 2018;175(2):103–11.

43. Al Sayegh A, Sandford D, Carson AJ. Psychological approaches to treatment of postconcussion syndrome: a systematic review. J Neurol Neurosurg Psychiatry 2010;81(10):1128–34.

44. Leddy JJ, Kozlowski K, Donnelly JP, et al. A preliminary study of subsymptom threshold exercise training for refractory post-concussion syndrome. Clin J Sport Med 2010;20(1):21–7.

45. Nelson LD, Tarima S, LaRoche AA, et al. Preinjury somatization symptoms contribute to clinical recovery after sport-related concussion. Neurology 2016; 86(20):1856–63.

46. Iverson GL, Gardner AJ, Terry DP, et al. Predictors of clinical recovery from concussion: a systematic review. Br J Sports Med 2017;51(12):941–8.

47. Ellis MJ, Leddy JJ, Willer B. Physiological, vestibulo-ocular and cervicogenic post-concussion disorders: an evidence-based classification system with directions for treatment. Brain Inj 2015;29(2):238–48.

48. Taylor DJ, Pruiksma KE. Cognitive and behavioural therapy for insomnia (CBT-I) in psychiatric populations: a systematic review. Int Rev Psychiatry 2014;26(2): 205–13.

49. DeMatteo C, Stazyk K, Giglia L, et al. A balanced protocol for return to school for children and youth following concussive injury. Clin Pediatr (Phila) 2015;54(8): 783–92.

50. McCrory P, Meeuwisse W, Dvořák J, et al. Consensus statement on concussion in sport-the 5. Br J Sports Med 2017;51(11):838–47.

51. Broglio SP, Cantu RC, Gioia GA, et al. National Athletic Trainers' Association position statement: management of sport concussion. J Athl Train 2014;49(2): 245–65.

Moving?

Make sure your subscription moves with you!

To notify us of your new address, find your **Clinics Account Number** (located on your mailing label above your name), and contact customer service at:

Email: journalscustomerservice-usa@elsevier.com

800-654-2452 (subscribers in the U.S. & Canada)
314-447-8871 (subscribers outside of the U.S. & Canada)

Fax number: 314-447-8029

Elsevier Health Sciences Division
Subscription Customer Service
3251 Riverport Lane
Maryland Heights, MO 63043

ELSEVIER

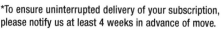

Printed and bound by CPI Group (UK) Ltd, Croydon, CR0 4YY

03/10/2024

01040403-0018